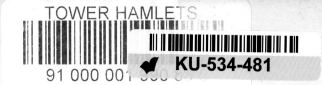

Understanding and dealing with
Depression

Foreword by Robbie Foy, Professor of Primary Care
at Leeds Institute of Health Sciences, University of Leeds

Dr Keith Souter WITHDRAWN

PERSONAL HEALTH GUIDES ✚

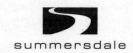

summersdale

UNDERSTANDING AND DEALING WITH DEPRESSION

Copyright © Keith Souter, 2013

Summersdale Publishers Ltd
46 West Street
Chichester
West Sussex
PO19 1RP
UK

www.summersdale.com

Printed and bound by CPI Group (UK) Ltd, Croydon, CR0 4YY

ISBN: 978-1-84953-391-1

Substantial discounts on bulk quantities of Summersdale books are available to corporations, professional associations and other organisations. For details contact Nicky Douglas by telephone: +44 (0) 1243 756902, fax: +44 (0) 1243 786300 or email: nicky@summersdale.com.

Disclaimer
Every effort has been made to ensure that the information in this book is accurate and current at the time of publication. The author and the publisher cannot accept responsibility for any misuse or misunderstanding of any information contained herein, or any loss, damage or injury, be it health, financial or otherwise, suffered by any individual or group acting upon or relying on information contained herein. None of the opinions or suggestions in this book are intended to replace medical opinion. If you have concerns about your health, please seek professional advice.

This book is dedicated to anyone who has ever experienced the oppressive burden of depression.

Acknowledgements

I would like to thank Isabel Atherton, my wonderful agent at Creative Authors, for helping to bring this book to light.

Thanks also to Claire Plimmer who commissioned the title and to Debbie Chapman, my project editor, whose suggestions have made this a better book than it otherwise would have been.

Thanks also to Rachael Wilkie, my copy-editor, who knocked some of the final rough edges off the manuscript.

It has been a pleasure to work with them all.

Finally, a big thank you to Professor Robbie Foy for taking the time out from his busy schedule to read the manuscript and write the foreword to this book.

Contents

Recognise that you need help
What you can do yourself

Chapter 10: Depression in children and young people

Changing society
Recognising depression in young people
Increased risk of depression in children and young people
Seeking help
Treatment available

Depression is not a normal part of getting old
How common is it?
Difficulty of diagnosis
Risk factors
Grief and depression
Dementia and depression
Diogenes syndrome
Iatrogenic depression
Psychosis in the elderly
Treatment of depression in the elderly
Help from family and neighbours

Baby blues
Postnatal depression
Risk factors for PND
Dealing with PND
Postpartum psychosis
Treatment of postpartum psychosis
Prognosis
Helpful organisations

It isn't getting any better
Antidepressants
Other treatments

Foreword

By Robbie Foy
Professor of Primary Care at Leeds Institute of Health Sciences, University of Leeds

For most of us, our lives have been affected by depression, be it through our own personal experience or contact with others. Some of us may have been affected without having realised it. About four out of five people with depression experience it more than once, and up to one in five experience it over many years. This common condition causes individual and family distress, dysfunction, and disability. It complicates other medical problems and causes many lost days of work.

So, what should we talk about when we talk about depression? Conversations with affected people and health professionals often cover three issues: recognising depression, seeking help, and coping and control.

Surprisingly for a condition with so many consequences, depression can be hard to recognise – by sufferers, friends and family, and health professionals. This is because it usually creeps up on people insidiously and changes how they feel, think and behave in a variety of ways. It may take some sort of personal crisis to make people realise that something is wrong. Its symptoms may not show in straightforward emotional ways; often people seek help for physical problems, such as sleep disturbance, chest pain or headaches. Detection can be especially difficult in those with long-term physical illnesses who are at greater risk of depression.

This is partly because its symptoms overlap with those of physical illness, such as fatigue in heart disease. However, one of the greatest barriers to recognition is the fear of having depression itself – people often worry that they will lose their jobs, lose their friends or lose their minds. People also see depression as something that happens to others and not to themselves. There is still a great deal of work to be done in challenging stigma and false beliefs about depression.

For those that seek professional help for depression, treatments available usually comprise antidepressant medication or talk therapy. As for many other aspects of healthcare, there are always new research findings to guide treatment decisions; these sometimes cause confusion. For example, family doctors in Britain used to be criticised for not prescribing antidepressants often enough and in high enough doses. It is now evident from research that antidepressants have limited effects on symptoms for people with less severe depression. Therefore, we are now seeing a continuing climb in antidepressant prescribing, which partly stems from professional habits and patient demand. The growing availability of talk therapies will hopefully provide people with depression with a greater choice of types of professional help. These treatment options do not undervalue the mainstay of treatment in British general practice: 'watchful waiting' combined with empathetic listening and support whilst people find their own paths to recovery.

People affected by depression also need to find their own ways to cope with symptoms and take back some control over their lives. This can be daunting, especially given that helplessness and loss of motivation typically go hand-in-hand with depression. Yet there is a wide range of practical measures. For example, what we do affects how we feel. It is worth identifying activities that someone with depression previously enjoyed but has missed since becoming depressed, and gradually taking them up again in small but steady steps. Everyday activities such as walking the dog or cooking can form part of a personal recovery or coping plan.

Dr Souter addresses such issues in this book, directly and with clarity. I hope that people will find it helpful in navigating through the often perplexing experience of depression safely and successfully.

Introduction

Most people will feel down in the dumps at some stage in their life. That is normal, and it is part and parcel of being human. Usually you can pinpoint the reason and relate it to some event in your life, or perhaps to something that has happened to a friend or relative. It may be to do with something that has happened at work, or even something that you have read about or seen on the television, which has stirred up a feeling of empathy. Such episodes normally do not last long and you can often rationalise the emotion and perhaps talk yourself out of it, or share it with a friend, finding that the feeling soon goes. Or you can distract yourself from it by doing something that you enjoy doing, and find that you soon get back to normal.

People can describe their feelings as being blue, sad, browned off, and so on. When we describe them in those terms, there is generally an acceptance that it is normal to experience such flattening of the spirits from time to time, and a tacit understanding that the feeling will not last long.

When these feelings last longer than a week or two, persisting for weeks on end and even for months, then that is quite different. So too is it different if the feeling is so bad that it begins to interfere with your life. This is likely to be actual depression. It is an indication that you need to do something about it and probably seek or mobilise help.

Depression is far more common than people imagine. According to the Office of National Statistics, one in ten of the adult population will be experiencing depression at any one time. Major depression, which we shall talk a lot about in this book, is occurring in one in twenty people at any one time. It is important to recognise this in yourself if you are feeling extremely low. If you ever think about harming yourself or have suicidal thoughts then you should seek help as soon as possible.

Depression is not a single entity. There are several forms of depression, which may need different approaches to manage them. It is important not to minimise the importance of adequately diagnosing and dealing with depression, because it is potentially a serious condition which can lead to self-harm of various sorts and even, in a small proportion of people, to genuine attempts at committing suicide.

Anxiety is also extremely common and many studies have shown that 70 per cent of people attending a GP's surgery will have anxiety as a component of their condition. The two conditions do co-exist, yet often an individual is not aware that they have the two problems. They may just feel that they are 'nervous', accepting a life filled with fear combined with long-standing flatness of mood as being their 'natural state'. But it does not have to be like this. If you can understand a bit more about what depression is and about how anxiety can mask it, then you can begin to take your feelings in hand so that you can enjoy life all the more.

The overall purpose of this book is to help you to understand depression and how it can affect you, or a relative or friend. It will also look at the various types of depression, the theories about what causes it and the different types of treatment and strategies that may help you deal with it. This will include support agencies and networks that are worth establishing to keep yourself depression-free.

The book naturally falls into three parts. Part One will look at the nature of depression, the different types and the theories that have been proposed, including current thought. Part Two will look at the different types of treatment, ranging from drug and physical treatments to the wide range of psychological and 'talking' therapies. Finally, Part Three will look at the various strategies, including nutrition, exercise and activities, that the individual can use to manage their own depression.

And so, to begin with, here are some general facts and figures about depression:

- Depression affects about 150 million people globally.

- Depression affects 1 in 5 people at some point in their life.

- At any time about 2.3 per cent of adults are depressed.

- Polls show that 60 per cent of people think that people with depression would be too embarrassed to consult their doctor.[1]

- 80 per cent of people with depression do not seek treatment.

- 8 per cent of the population suffer from mixed anxiety and depression.

- The lifetime risk of developing depression is 8 per cent for men.

- The lifetime risk of developing depression is 12 per cent for women

- About 8 per cent of children and adolescents under the age of 15 years suffer from depression.

- There are around 4,000 suicides per year in the UK – 70 per cent of these are people who were depressed.

- Between 2 and 9 per cent of people with depression will commit suicide.[2]

- It takes on average 10 years and £350 million to develop a new antidepressant.

- The global drug market for psychotropic medication in 2012 was estimated at $15 billion.

PART ONE

UNDERSTANDING DEPRESSION

In this section, we are going to look at what depression feels like and consider the difficulty that doctors and patients have had over the years in trying to understand this very distressing condition. Some people may have a very clear reason why they have become depressed and they may well benefit from one of the various types of talking therapy. Others may have no reason why they should feel so flat and down. Their problem may be to do with brain chemistry and the levels of their neurotransmitters. It is possible that they may benefit from taking antidepressants.

Yet it is not always as clear-cut as that. The choice of treatment is sometimes very difficult. It all relates to how well the individual's depression is understood, by themselves as well as by healthcare professionals.

Chapter 1

What do we mean by depression?

Even a happy life cannot be without a measure of darkness, and the word 'happy' would lose its meaning if it were not balanced by sadness.

Carl Jung (1875–1961), psychologist and psychiatrist

Emotions and thoughts

Emotions are strange things. Philosophers have wondered about their purpose for eons. If we human beings were simply hard thinking, logical, unemotional creatures, wouldn't life be simpler? If we had no emotions, then perhaps decisions could be based on logic alone, devoid of sentiments that colour our judgement. Similarly, we might be spared the grief of bereavements, the sorrow of parting with loved ones and the anxiety that certain situations cause us. And how much pleasanter it would be if we were not subject to anger, jealousy or sadness.

On the other hand, if we had no emotions it might be hard to appreciate life, since the aesthetics – the finer things like beauty, music and our ability to suspend belief when we watch a film or read a novel – would be impaired. We would not experience the joy of hearing a joke, or seeing a child play, or upon receiving a pleasant surprise. And perhaps our emotions are important in decision making, especially if a decision calls for us to empathise with someone and act in a caring manner.

Having thoughts and experiencing emotions are both things that characterise us, and the two are often interlinked. Few people are capable of cold, clinical, unemotional thoughts. You may be able to suspend your emotions in a professional situation, for example, when you know what you need to do or how to behave in a particular manner in keeping with your occupation. Yet you cannot do it throughout your whole life. Your emotions will affect your thinking at some times of the day in some ways. The fact is, like it or not, those emotions do tend to make you think differently.

Sometimes, for no obvious reason, you may wake up feeling in a sombre mood. You just feel flat. As a result, you will tend to approach the day in a different manner from a day on which you wake up feeling it is a pleasure to be alive. Your thoughts may be guided or swayed by that feeling. You may think in a negative manner, and follow a negative line of thought that makes you adopt particular behaviours. For example, you may normally be able to control a particular habit, such as drinking alcohol, when you are feeling well and feeling positive. When you are feeling negative, your resistance may weaken and you indulge in the habit, which in turn may induce other emotions, like guilt or anger, further intensifying the negativity. On the other hand, when you are feeling joyful and positive you may see humour in things, you may feel more confident to perform certain tasks and you may adopt behaviours compatible with that mood.

These are simple examples of the way that emotions may colour our thoughts. Similarly, by thinking in a particular way you can generate different types of emotion. You can talk yourself into getting angry, or jealous or sad.

Undoubtedly, some emotions, like happiness or pity, are useful as they prompt us to act in an appropriate manner. In this they can be compared with the sensation of pain, which compels us to act in a way which will lessen the pain or remove its cause.

Unfortunately, other emotions seem to be simply destructive and unneccessary. They do not help us, they do not make us feel good, they just make us feel bad in some way.

Depression is such a feeling.

Just feeling down or feeling depressed

Feeling down or sad is a common and normal experience. Most people will experience it in certain situations, for example when something unfortunate occurs in their life or in the life of someone close to them. It is usually a fairly transient feeling, however, that rarely lasts longer than a week or two.

Depression, on the other hand, is a lot more intense and it lasts for longer. It may go on for weeks or months. In addition, the feelings in depression are so intense that they actually interfere with life. They may make it hard to get any pleasure from anything.

Sufferers describe it as feeling stuck in a deep hole with no way out, or as if they are living in a grey world with no colour, or simply existing in a joyless world.

The sufferer's image of themselves is also usually affected. They may dislike themselves, or feel that they are useless, of little or no value and even that they are unlovable.

And sometimes people can feel so bad and so unhappy that they feel their life has no meaning. They may even think of self-harm.

KEY POINTS

- In depression the mood is low or flat for weeks or months rather than days.
- In depression the feelings are so bad that they interfere with one's life.

How do you know if you are depressed?

Unlike your general health where your doctor can perform various blood tests to assess your state of wellbeing, in depression there is no clear blood test, no neurotransmitter level that can be assessed. Depression is all about how you feel.

If someone thinks that they might be depressed it is important to do something about it. There is always something that can be done to help or someone who can help.

Answering the following basic questions may give an indication:

Do you feel unhappy most days?

Have you lost interest in life and find yourself unable to enjoy anything?

Do you feel low in the morning, but better in the evening?

Do you feel indifferent to everyone?

Do you feel so bad at times that you just want to run away?

Do you avoid people or situations?

Do you have difficulty concentrating on things that you normally handle with ease?

Have you lost your confidence?

Do you find it hard to make decisions?

Do you feel bad about yourself?

Do you ever feel that you are a failure, or think that you are useless or of no value?

Do you feel guilty about something?

Do you have difficulty with your sleep?

Do you get irritable or angry?

Do you cry for no reason?

Do you feel excessively tired, so that some days you cannot achieve anything?

Have you lost your appetite and started to lose weight?

Have you found yourself comfort-eating and putting weight on?

Have you lost your sex drive or had problems with your sex life?

Do you have a bleak view of your future?

Have you thought of self-harming?

Have you ever thought about committing suicide?

These are actually the sort of questions that a doctor will ask you. Some questions are of more significance than others. The first two in particular are the cornerstones of the diagnosis. So if the answer is 'yes' to those two and several more, all of them having lasted for more than two weeks, that suggests that depression is present.

TAKE THE QUESTIONNAIRE

The questions laid out here are very general. If you find that you answer yes to five or six then you may be depressed. Many more than that, you could be suffering quite badly. If so, in Chapter 6 you can find a self-administered questionnaire called the Patient Health Questionnaire, which is used as a diagnostic aid. Turn to p.72 if you would like to check now.

KEY POINTS

Two key features of depression are:

- Feeling continuously unhappy for two weeks or more
- Having lost interest and enjoyment of life for two weeks or more

Depression may be hidden

People very often do not accept that they are depressed. They may take the view that depression is something that happens to other people. Or they may not believe that it exists. Or they may even believe that it is a form of mental weakness and that they could not possibly admit to anyone that they were feeling down and depressed, for fear that they would be considered weak.

The fact is that there is still a social stigma against depression. Even today, in our so-called enlightened times, people do believe that being diagnosed with depression could affect their work, their chance of getting a loan, a mortgage or medical insurance. The embarrassment that people have can be so strong that it prevents them from seeking help even though they would benefit immensely from it. Polls show that about 60 per cent of the adult population feel that people with depression would be too embarrassed to see a doctor. In fact, 80 per cent of people who are depressed do not seek help. That means they are suffering in silence.

In some people, depression can manifest in physical symptoms such as chronic headaches, abdominal pains or various painful conditions, often causing a vicious circle to develop. Depression can underlie a problem, but the negative feelings that are then associated with the symptoms can worsen the depression. In that case, treating the depression may help to alleviate or even cure the physical problems.

KEY POINTS

- Depression is not a form of mental weakness. It should be regarded in the same way as any other symptom, such as pain.
- Depression may cause other problems, such as insomnia or chronic physical complaints.

A problem shared is a problem halved

This old adage has a lot of truth in it. Sometimes, the simple act of confiding in a friend or relative about a problem can remove the anxiety associated with it. Essentially, unburdening yourself can help in that the person you confide in may be able to offer advice, empathy and support.

If the depression is not alleviated by this, it may be that further support and help is needed, possibly from your doctor.

When you should seek help

You may not feel like burdening a friend or relative and feel instead that you can just soldier on. However, ask yourself why you should just go on suffering. You may find that you will be able to function better and be, for example, a better friend, partner or parent if you seek help. Quite simply, the sooner you seek aid the sooner you are likely to feel better.

There are generally four situations which are strong indications that you need help.

These are:

If your feelings of depression are persisting and not getting better, or they are getting worse.

If your depressed mood is affecting your life. That effect can be in relation to family and social life, work, or leisure.

If you start having morbid thoughts and feel useless and of no value.

If you contemplate or cannot stop thinking about self-harming or suicide.

Chapter 2

The causes of depression

In sooth, I know not why I am so sad:
It wearies me; you say it wearies you;
But how I caught it, found it, or came by it,
What stuff 'tis made of, whereof it is born,
I am to learn;
And such a want-wit sadness makes of me,
That I have much ado to know myself.

William Shakespeare (1564–1616) *The Merchant of Venice*,
Act 1, Scene 1

Cause unknown!

William Shakespeare, the great English playwright, knew a great deal about depression. Indeed, within his plays he gives us studies of all of the emotions, including jealousy, anger, guilt and depression. In his day, it was called melancholy, and he has many characters describe so eloquently what it feels like to be melancholic, or depressed. In the above quotation from the very first speech in the first scene of his play, *The Merchant of Venice*, the character Antonio introduces himself with a confession that he is depressed. The lines tell us that, although he recognises how melancholic he feels, he cannot understand the reasons why.

That is a common experience in depression. People often do not know why they have become depressed. It is almost as if a dark curtain of gloom descends upon them and they cannot lift it.

Just because you don't know why you are feeling depressed does not mean that you are not depressed, or that you should feel embarrassed about seeking help. If you are feeling depressed, then it is certainly worth seeking help – the sooner the better.

Famous people who have suffered from depression

Depression is no respector of persons. Many famous people throughout history have experienced depression:

Michelangelo (1475–1564) – Italian sculptor and artist

Sir Isaac Newton (1642–1727) – English mathematician and physicist, discoverer of gravity

Hans Christian Andersen (1805–1875) – Danish writer of fairy tales

Raymond Chandler (1888–1959) – American crime writer and screenwriter

Agatha Christie (1890–1976) – English crime writer

Charles Dickens (1812–1870) – English novelist

T. S. Eliot (1888–1965) – American poet, publisher and playwright

Winston Churchill (1874–1965) – writer, politician, former Prime Minister of the UK

Paul Gauguin (1848–1903) – French artist

Sylvia Plath (1932–1963) – American writer and poet

And many celebrities today have admitted to suffering from depression:

Ian Thorpe – five time Olympic champion swimmer

Brad Pitt – American actor and movie star

Angelina Jolie – American actress

Catherine Zeta Jones – Welsh actress

Stephen Fry – English actor, playwright and author

Paul Merton – English comedian

Marie Osmond – American singer

Anne Rice – American writer

Uma Thurman – American actress

Owen Wilson – American actor and screenwriter

Some causes of depression

Although Shakespeare has Antonio say that he does not know why he feels so melancholic, for many people there will be a recognisable cause or a trigger. Sometimes, there may be several factors that all contribute to making you feel depressed. A life event may have had a significant effect on your circumstances and you may have developed a habit to make you feel better, such as having a drink. That may have escalated and caused you to isolate yourself from friends and family and depression may be triggered.

The following may be potential causes:

Stressful event

A bereavement, a relationship break-up, divorce, a traumatic event affecting your health, a move of house, a sudden financial problem, and so on. All of these things create stress and it is normal that they take time to settle down. In some people, the event itself can be enough to cause depression, or it could be a triggering factor if there are other stresses that are having to be dealt with.

Personal circumstances

Loneliness and isolation for one reason or another often make us more vulnerable. This is understandable, since they mean that you feel like you have no one to share problems with or discuss how you feel.

Financial difficulty is another perfectly understandable problem that can be very stressful and contribute to depression. It can be hard to stop thinking about such problems.

Physical illness

Some physical illnesses can have a profound effect on your circumstances. If you are no longer able to work then financial difficulties may ensue.

Some conditions put you at a higher risk of developing depression, especially life-threatening ones like heart disease and cancer. They affect you physically *and* emotionally, since your life may be altered dramatically. You may feel anxiety about the future and depression because you are more aware of your mortality.

Some conditions such as hypothyroidism (underactive thyroid gland) and chronic fatigue syndrome, which may make the sufferer feel very tired and fatigued, are also associated with low mood. Not having the energy to do the things that you want to do can contribute to depression.

Chronic painful conditions, like arthritis, chronic back pain or facial neuralgia, may make life so difficult to cope with that a downward spiral into depression is not uncommon.

Some people become quite depressed if they contract viral infections, such as glandular fever which mainly affects young adults.

Other severe infections, like pneumonia, recurrent urinary infections, or an attack of shingles can affect older adults and may cause depression.

Personality

Some people seem to be more prone to depression. Their outlook upon life may be pessimistic and they may find it difficult to be positive about the future. This could be due to events that took place in their childhood or in their past.

Family

If several people in the family have suffered with depression in the past then it may suggest that an individual will be more at risk of becoming depressed.

Again, this may have its origins in the dynamics that operate within the family. On the other hand it may be that there is a genetic predisposition to depression. It is hard to be precise, since it is the old question of nature or nurture. Whatever the case may be, if a family member has suffered from depression then there is an increased risk that other family members may also be prone to depression.

The diathesis-stress theory of depression is the name given to the nature or nurture question. We shall consider it in **Chapter 4, Theories of depression**.

KEY POINT

- If a parent had depression then there is an eightfold increase in the risk that the children will develop depression at some point in their lives

Gender

Women are more prone to depression than men. The lifetime risk of developing depression is 8 per cent for men, compared with 12 per cent for women.

Why this should be the case is unclear, although it is possible that many of the men who suffer from depression are hidden. Instead of talking about it and acknowledging that there is a problem, they may be more likely to drink, become aggressive or adopt other behaviour patterns.

This is very worrying, as men tend not to seek help from their doctor for many things as often as women. The social stigma that we discussed earlier may have a lot to do with this, in that men may feel that it is not macho to admit to having sad feelings, and certainly not depression. The fact that three times more men than women commit suicide may indicate that men are more likely to avoid treatment and suffer in silence.

Alcohol and drug abuse

People often resort to alcohol and other recreational drugs to help them deal with a situation. The tendency may then be to develop a dependence, which brings with it all the other problems of alcohol and drug abuse. This is a strong risk factor for depression.

People who experiment with drugs are at high risk of developing an addiction. Even if you only use 'soft' drugs such as cannabis, the truth is that you are not safe. These drugs interfere with neurotransmitters (the natural messenger chemicals that are involved in the transmission of signals along nerves and between brain cells) and there is strong evidence that they can provoke anxiety and depression. There is also mounting evidence that they can provoke serious psychiatric problems such as schizophrenic psychosis in some individuals.

Iatrogenic depression

This means depression caused by treatment. The term comes from the Greek words *iatros*, meaning 'doctor', and *gen*, meaning 'made by'. It is depression caused by drugs prescribed for other things. The drugs listed below all have depression as a potential side effect.

DRUGS THAT MAY CAUSE IATROGENIC DEPRESSION

Accutane – a drug used to treat severe acne.

Acyclovir – a drug used to treat shingles.

Antabuse – a drug used to treat alcoholism.

Anticonvulsants – there are several drugs used to treat epilepsy that can cause depression, including methsuximide and ethosuximide.

Antipsychotic drugs – drugs used to manage psychosis.

Barbiturates – these are anti-anxiety drugs, which were used until the newer benzodiazepine group of anti-anxiety drugs were introduced. Some, such as phenobarbitone, are still used in epilepsy.

Beta-blockers – these are commonly used to treat various heart conditions and hypertension.

Bromocriptine – used to treat Parkinson's disease.

Calcium-channel blockers – these are commonly used to treat certain heart conditions and in hypertension.

Hormone Replacement Therapy – can sometimes cause depression.

Levo-dopa – a drug used to treat Parkinson's disease.

Opiates – used in the control of severe pain.

Oral contraceptive pill – a study by the Alfred Psychiatry Research Centre in Australia in 2005 showed a link between several types of contraceptive pill and depression.[3]

Statins – used to control cholesterol.

Steroids – used to treat inflammation and inflammatory conditions.

If depression is caused by any of these drugs then it should settle simply by withdrawing the drug. This should only be done with your doctor's approval. You should never suddenly stop taking a drug without consulting your doctor, since some may be associated with a rebound effect and the withdrawal may need to be done slowly.

Advancing age

Depression in the elderly is often missed. It can often be so severe that it is mistaken for the early signs of dementia. We shall return to this in **Chapter 11, Depression in older age**.

Postnatal depression

Some women are prone to becoming depressed after they have given birth. This is something that has been recognised for centuries rather than being a condition that has developed in modern society.

The condition seems to happen to women who are predisposed to depression and is thought to be a result of the monumental changes that take place in their physiology during pregnancy and following childbirth. We shall return to this subject in Chapter 12.

Chapter 3

The types of depression

Knowing your own darkness is the best method for dealing with the darknesses of other people.

Carl Jung (1875–1961), psychologist and psychiatrist

As we saw in the last chapter, there are many potential causes of depression which seem to just descend without reason and without any obvious trigger. Yet depression does not come in just one form; there are many distinct types, which doctors have attempted to classify over the years. It was thought that by diagnosing specific types of depression, it would be possible to predict the way the disease would develop and how best to treat it.

That has been the aim, but the truth is that it is a highly controversial area. Different classification systems have been offered over the years and then modified. It is worth looking at the systems that have been used in the past, because they all have merits as well as certain disadvantages. By considering them, we will then see why the classification that is used today is now accepted to be the most useful.

Older classifications

In the next chapter, when we come to look at the various theories about the mechanism of depression, we shall see that it is a very complex area. There are physical theories that relate to the way in which the brain works, psychodynamic theories that relate to the way the mind is thought to work, and there are behavioural theories that look at the ways in which one's behaviour can affect one's emotions and vice versa.

These different schools of thought have led to different views about how depression should be and can be treated. And those ideas led to the classifications that were used up until relatively recently.

Neurotic and psychotic depression

These two terms were first introduced in the mid-nineteenth century. It was believed that neurotic depression was neurologically based, hence the 'neuro' prefix, because people often also suffered from physical symptoms. That is, anxiety was often a component of the depression and the individual might describe palpitations, perspiration or abdominal cramps associated with their mood changes. It was thought that this was a lesser type of problem than psychotic depression.

Psychotic depression was thought to be a disturbance of the mind, to the extent that the individual could lose touch with reality. Sometimes the individual would, in addition to the low mood, suffer from hallucinations and delusions.

A delusion is a false belief that cannot be rationalised and that the individual cannot be talked out of. A hallucination is an impression that something is happening which in reality is not. Seeing angels or people when there is no one present is an example of a visual hallucination, and hearing voices instructing you to do something is an example of an auditory hallucination.

In lay terms, these two types would equate with 'nerves' and 'madness'.

It was felt that neurosis could be treated with talking therapies and antidepressants, while psychotic depression would need much stronger treatment with powerful drugs called antipsychotics and electro-convulsive therapy (ECT).

The great problem with this classification is that very often in severe depression there will be no hallucinations or delusions. It is also possible that to be labelled 'psychotic' could have a stigma and other implications regarding work and insurance.

For these reasons this classification is discouraged and is no longer used.

Endogenous and reactive depression

These terms were regularly used when I worked in psychiatry early in my career. They relate to the supposed cause of the depression.

Endogenous, from the Greek *endon*, meaning 'within', was thought to be depression that was the result of genes or biochemical changes within the brain. It was to do with the individual's internal workings and their inherited tendencies. The symptoms of depression would include so-called 'biological' features that indicated changes in the way that the body worked. Hence there could be weight loss, loss of appetite, sleep disturbance (in that one would wake early in the morning) and diurnal variation (a tendency to feel most depressed at the start of the day, but gradually improving as the day went on).

Reactive or 'exogenous' depression, from the Latin *ex*, meaning 'out', was thought to be a result of a reaction to something in the individual's life, such as a grief reaction, or a reaction to loss or some trauma. There would be more anxiety symptoms and the sleep disturbance would be difficulty falling asleep rather than waking early, as with endogenous depression. This was thought to be a more understandable form of depression and to be less severe.

Endogenous depression was said to be amenable to physical treatments and drugs.

Reactive depression was said to improve with reassurance, time and perhaps on-going support and talking treatment. It was felt that these patients probably would not respond to antidepressants.

The problems with older classifications

There are similarities between these two classifications. Neurotic depression has similarities with reactive depression, and psychotic depression has some similarities with endogenous depresion. However, the difficulty with them lies in the fact that people who are depressed often have multiple factors that may fit one or both. Someone who seemingly has an endogenous depression, for example, may have a triggering traumatic event, which would also be in keeping with the reactive pattern.

There is no blood test or instrumental reading that can differentiate whether a depression is biochemical or psychodynamic. The problem is that the assessment of how one feels is totally subjective. In other words, only the individual can know what they feel. A doctor or therapist cannot actually get inside the depressed person's mind and the best they can do is make a decision based upon what their patient has told them. But, very importantly, at a practical level the two types cannot be readily divided into those who will or will not respond to drug treatment. The margins are really quite blurred.

The current classification

Nowadays, it is recognised that it is difficult to be precise about how we categorise depression. What is helpful is in trying to ask a number of questions in order to work out how severe the depression is.

Primary or secondary

In order to determine whether depression is primary or secondary, a doctor will ask if the symptoms are the result of any physical or psychological condition. If the answer is 'No', then the depression is said to be primary.

If the answer is 'Yes', then the depression is secondary to that condition. The treatment should aim to deal with the condition that the depression is secondary to.

There is actually no hard evidence to distinguish these from each other. The point is really that if an underlying cause can be found, for example an underactive thyroid gland, or a chronic medical condition, or iatrogenic depression (drug-induced depression, see Chapter 2) then there is a treatment target.

Severity

This can be difficult for an individual to self-assess, because when you are feeling depressed it can be impossible to quantify. Even if the person is not suffering from many symptoms of depression, they may feel desperate.

Rather, the assessment relates to how incapacitating their case is. We therefore divide depression into three categories:

- *Mild depression* – where the depression does not stop the person with getting on with their daily life. They probably find it hard, but they cope. In mild depression the person may respond to talking therapies and will probably not be prescribed antidepressant medication. Counselling may be suggested.

- *Moderate depression* – where the depression impacts on daily life and there is an increase in symptoms of depression. The person is probably able to cope at some level, but is struggling, and on some days is not able to cope. In moderate depression the person may very well be prescribed antidepressant medication and probably also counselling or other talking therapy.

- *Severe depression* – where the depression is so bad that the person has no interest in anything and finds it impossible to function. Even eating and sleeping may seem impossible and there may be no interest in getting out of bed. There may be a real risk of self-harm or thoughts of suicide. In severe depression the person will almost certainly be prescribed antidepressants and probably also talking therapies.

- *Psychotic depression* – 10–15 per cent of people with severe depression may experience hallucinations and delusions, disturbance of thought and confusion and reduced awareness or insight. In particular, they may have paranoid delusions when they think that people are talking about them or conspiring against them. Some people can develop grandiose ideas. They may be exceedingly irritable and angry and neglectful of themselves. If they do have insight that their delusions are not real then they may be ashamed of them and try to hide them or not express them to others. This can make diagnosis difficult.

- They usually need hospital treatment and may require antipsychotic medication, mood stabilisers and antidepressants. If medication does not work then ECT may be needed. Generally, however, the prognosis is very good and it can be cured, although regular follow-ups will always be needed.

The differentiation into the three types of depression is made on the basis of the presence of depressive symptoms, as outlined in Chapter 1, and the method of assessing may use the Patient Health Questionnaire in Chapter 6. The severity of the symptoms is also taken into account. The three typical symptoms of depression are:

- Depressed mood
- Loss of interest and enjoyment of life
- Reduced energy.

Symptoms are typically thought significant if they persevere for a period of two weeks or more.

For a diagnosis of mild depression, two of the typical symptoms and two other symptoms indicate depression.

For a diagnosis of moderate depression, two of the typical symptoms plus three other symptoms are needed.

For a diagnosis of severe depression, all three of the typical symptoms are needed and at least four other symptoms.

Specific types of depression

There are, however, several other types of depression that require separate consideration.

Unipolar depression

This is not different from the three types of depression, but refers to the pattern of depression that a person may have. It is the diagnosis given when a person has had several episodes of depression. It is only ever depressed mood that they experience, rather than elevated mood or mania. The treatments that they get will be talking therapies or antidepressants. It tends to affect about 7 per cent of the adult population. It typically occurs in the 30–40 age group.

Bipolar depression

This used to be called manic-depression. It tends to be a severer form than unipolar. The person experiences episodes of extreme depression followed by episodes of mania. One episode of mania is needed to make this diagnosis. Three or four episodes per year may occur.

The manic phases are typified by increased energy, pressure of speech so that the person fills the air with words, and pressure of thought so that they flit from idea to idea, leaving things unfinished. They may be unable to concentrate, their minds jumping from one subject to the next. There may be a highly elevated mood, bizarre or even aggressive behaviour and denial that there is anything wrong.

This affects 2–3 per cent of the population. It may be associated with delusions of grandeur amongst others, and sometimes by hallucinations. It typically starts earlier than unipolar depression, sometimes in the person's 20s.

There is a higher risk of suicide with bipolar depression than with any other form of depression.

It is important to differentiate between unipolar depression and bipolar depression, since the treatments needed are different. Bipolar depression may be worsened by the use of antidepressants, which can actually provoke an episode of mania. It may be more effectively treated with a mood-stabilising drug such as lithium, valproate or lamotrigine.

Dysthymia

This is not so much an illness, more a permanently flattened mood. It affects about 2 per cent of the population.

It is characterised by low mood, but it does not interfere with the person's life. They can function and cope, but always feel they do so below par.

In terms of diagnosis, there will be one or two of the depressive symptoms but they tend not to be severe. They are present for in excess of two years and they may be more marked at times and may even disappear for short spells.

Antidepressants may work, but they take longer to work than they do in depression. Talking therapies are more likely to benefit someone with dysthymia. If it is diagnosed then it is as well to keep on top of it, since people with dysthymia are more at risk of developing a full-blown depression.

Some patients with dysthymia also experience major or severe depression at the same time. That is, they are feeling depressed, then swing into a severe depression for a while before returning to their usual milder dysthymia. This is called double depression. If this happens then it is important to see your doctor for a fresh assessment and treatment.

Postnatal depression

It is normal to feel a bit down after giving birth and about 60–70 per cent of new mothers experience this. In about 13 per cent of new mothers this feeling is far more severe and does not lift. It is typified by ongoing feelings of sadness, fatigue, loneliness, feeling unable to cope, and feeling unworthy. There may also be thoughts of suicide or fears of hurting the baby. Rather distressingly for all concerned, there may be a feeling that the mother cannot bond with her child. At its worst, she may even reject the child.

It can occur anywhere from a few weeks to a few months after birth. Treatment may necessitate both talking therapy and drugs treatment. We shall consider this at greater length in **Chapter 12, Postnatal depression**.

Seasonal Affective Disorder

Some people seem to become depressed during the winter months and almost seem to want to hibernate. They may gain weight, withdraw from friends and family and experience mild to moderate depression. They also tend to become more anxious and irritable.

Seasonal Affective Disorder, or SAD, affects about 5 per cent of the adult population. It is thought that it relates to the reduction in light exposure. It starts in early winter and lifts in the spring.

It often responds to getting up, being outside as much as one can to get the light and also by using an artificial light box. These are boxes containing intense bright light, which the SAD sufferer sits in front of for a session each day. Light intensity is measured in lux. An ordinary lightbulb will only give out 200–500 lux, whereas a light therapy box will give out at least 2,500 lux. A session of 30–45 minutes may be enough to see a significant improvement.

Atypical depression

The very name of this implies that it is not like the description of depression that we have seen so far throughout this book. In fact, it is really very common.

It typically causes a feeling of heaviness, as if the arms and legs feel inordinately heavy. There is also a tendency to overeat, oversleep and overreact and be irritable. The individual may not be aware that they are depressed until they are questioned about it.

Talking therapies may help considerably.

Situational depression

This is the type of depression that follows an obvious trigger, such as bereavement, losing one's job or having a relationship break-up. It tends to produce a minor depression. Reassurance and support are usually all that is needed and drug treatment is not usually required.

This is not to trivialise it, however, since if one does experience such an episode which seems to be taking a long time to clear, it can lapse into a more severe depression needing more intensive treatment.

Premenstrual Dysphoric Disorder

About 75 per cent of women experience some degree of premenstrual syndrome, which usually affects them in the week before their period is due and causes weepiness, irritability or mood swings. Five per cent of women experience an actual depression with anxiety and severe mood swings, sometimes so extreme that they have angry and even violent outbursts that they cannot control.

These can affect the sufferer's relationships at work and at home and indeed can cause problems in any social situation if a temper tantrum or weepiness is triggered. Treatment with hormones, drugs or nutritional advice (see Chapter 15) may be needed.

Grief reaction

To grieve after the loss of someone important in your life is normal. In some people, the normal bereavement reaction is prolonged leading to a severe depression. It can be very troublesome and is often associated with thoughts of self-harm. It may require drugs and talking therapies.

The Mental Health Act

The Mental Health Act of 1983 is the law, relevant in England and Wales, that allows people with a mental disorder to be admitted, detained and treated in hospital without their consent. This is used if it is considered that the person is either a danger to themselves or to other people. It was amended in 2007 and again amended by the introduction of the Health and Social Care Act of 2012.

The majority of people treated in psychiatric hospitals are admitted informally, meaning they are admitted with their own consent. About 25 per cent of people are admitted by being 'sectioned' under the Mental Health Act. This means that they have been detained under one of the sections of the Act. They are formal patients and this means that they cannot leave during the time allowed by the relevant section.

Two doctors will examine and assess the patient to confirm that such detainment is appropriate and necessary.

If someone is detained under the Act then they should take legal advice to ensure that the exact processes have been followed.

More information can be obtained from the Department of Health website: www.dh.gov.uk/health/2012/06/act-explained/

Chapter 4

Theories about depression

There is no greater cause of melancholy than idleness, 'no better cure than business', as Rhasis holds.

Robert Burton (1576–1640), *The Anatomy of Melancholy*

The humoral theory of the ancient Greeks

The old name for depression was melancholia or melancholy. It is an archaic term that goes right back to the days of the father of medicine, Hippocrates of Cos, who practised medicine in the mid-fifth century BC. The word comes from the Greek words *melas*, meaning 'black' and *chole*, meaning 'bile'. It literally means black bile, and Hippocrates taught that an excess of this caused the depression in spirits – hence it came to mean 'sadness'.

The Doctrine of Humors was the theory that dominated medical thought for most of the next two millennia, until the Renaissance, which stated that there were four fundamental humors, or body fluids, which determined the state of health of the individual: blood, yellow bile, black bile and phlegm. It was thought that the humors were associated with the four elements – air, fire, earth and water – which in turn were paired with certain qualities: hot, cold, dry and moist. Thus, earth would be dry and cold, water would be wet and cold, fire would be hot and dry, and air would be wet and hot.

A condition would be diagnosed and formulated as being due to excess or deficiency of one or other humor and treatment would aim at removing the excess or giving a medicine which would boost it.

In the case of melancholia, Hippocrates taught that it was caused by an excess of black bile, hence the name. A person who had a tendency to bouts of melancholia was described as melancholic.

Rhazes, the great Persian physician

Muhammad ibn Zakariya al-Razi (865–925) was a Persian polymath. He was a philosopher, physician, alchemist and scholar, who made important contributions to several fields of knowledge. He became world famous under the Latinised name of Rhasis or Rhazes.

As a scientist, he questioned the humoral theory and modified it to include the concept that mental illness and melancholia in some cases could be attributed to the patient's possession by demons. Severe melancholia could result in false and wild thinking (hallucinations and delusions), which indicated that the thoughts were not the individual's own but those of the possessing demons.

Despite this clear misconception, he did have useful ideas about how to treat melancholia. He advocated distracting the mind, as in the quote by the Jacobean scholar Robert Burton at the start of this chapter. He also suggested the use of prescriptions of the poppy or its juice, which of course we now call opium, and *Cuscuta epithymium*, or clover dodder.

He was also the first doctor to try to make medicines easier to take by mixing them into small balls, which were wrapped in very fine silver foil. Effectively, he helped to develop the pill as a means of taking medication. For that alone, many patients would have been grateful, since many of the potions and nostrums used until then would have been stomach churning.

The Anatomy of Melancholy

Robert Burton was an Oxford scholar and vicar who suffered from melancholia, or depression. He had studied the works of Rhazes and absorbed much of the ideas about melancholia. Indeed, in an attempt to deal with his own state of mind he wrote a six-volume work entitled *The Anatomy of Melancholy* in 1621. He was quite candid about his reasons for writing it: 'I write of melancholy by being busy to avoid melancholy.'

The work was the first real and useful book on psychiatry. It covered the subject from the viewpoints of astrology, medicine, philosophy and proto-psychology. In it, he produced a model of consciousness and a model of the mind which, although now seen as flawed, nevertheless gave a framework with which people could work. Its influence lasted for at least two centuries and it remains a fascinating classic of Renaissance literature.

He described a melancholic disposition, or tendency to melancholia, as:

Melancholy, the subject of our present discourse, is either in disposition or in habit. In disposition, is that transitory

> *Melancholy* which goes and comes upon every small occasion of sorrow, need, sickness, trouble, fear, grief, passion, or perturbation of the mind, any manner of care, discontent, or thought, which causes anguish, dullness, heaviness and vexation of spirit, any ways opposite to pleasure, mirth, joy, delight, causing forwardness in us, or a dislike.

And he differentiated it from melancholia as an illness, which could be acquired as a habit:

> *Melancholy* of which we are to treat, is a habit, a serious ailment, a settled humour, as Aurelianus and others call it, not errant, but fixed: and as it was long increasing, so, now being (pleasant or painful) grown to a habit, it will hardly be removed.

Burton described 'causeless melancholia', the type that descends upon a sufferer for no reason, much as Shakespeare had described it in the character of Antonio in his play *The Merchant of Venice*. He advised that people with melancholia could be helped by getting good sleep, eating healthily, and by being distracted by listening to music and talking with good friends.

Nineteenth century – the beginning of psychiatry

Science and medicine really began to advance in the nineteenth century and several doctors attempted to differentiate between the types of melancholia.

Dr Emil Kraepelin (1856–1926), the father of psychiatry, described *involutional melancholia* as a state of depression at the menopause, from the Latin *involvere*, the process of enfolding or returning. His belief was that the uterus was shrinking and returning to its immature, infertile state.

In 1870, Dr Henry Maudsley (1835-1918) wrote *Body and Mind: An Inquiry into their Connection and Mutual Influence*, one of the first texts to try to understand the nature of the mind in sickness and in health. In 1907, he founded the world-famous Maudsley Hospital in London (finally opened in 1923) for the care of people with mental and emotional problems.

Twentieth-century theories

The twentieth century saw the development of several streams of practice in psychology (the study of the mind) and psychiatry (the medical treatment of mental disorders). Each of these offered plausible theories about depression.

Psychodynamic theories

Essentially, psychodynamic theories have been based upon the works of several early thinkers, who all developed their own system of therapy. They all consider that emotional problems stem from unconscious mental processes.

Sigmund Freud and psychoanalysis

Freud was a neurologist who developed a model of the mind that was based on the medical model. According to his theory, the psyche consists of:

• The super-ego, the controller of the mind, which acts as the individual's conscience.

- The id, the unconscious instinctive and self-gratifying part that is like a mischievous little child.

- The ego, or the conscious, which is the projection of the self, after integrating the drive of the id and the strictures of the super-ego.

Freud developed the process of psychoanalysis by free association which works by allowing free thoughts to be expressed and the individual helped to recognise their symbolism in order to resolve conflicts in the mind.

Freud postulated that depression relates to loss. This can be triggered by any kind of loss, whether it is of a person, a thing, or a status. This loss can be internalised into a feeling of rejection, which can produce self-hatred. The individual then starts to self-loathe and becomes depressed. As the process develops, the person believes that they are responsible for the symbolic loss, whatever it actually was. This causes lack of confidence, and loss of self-esteem.

This can all relate, according to Freud, to the relationship with one's parents in early life. If the person does not have positive feelings about those early relationships, then there may be a predisposition towards depression, which can be triggered by the symbolic loss.

Carl Jung and Jungian analysis
Jung explained depression in terms of his libido theory. By libido, he meant psychic energy. He did not necessarily consider depression to be a bad thing, or an illness that needed to be treated and removed or suppressed, but a state that needed to be understood. If the symptom could be understood, then it would be reduced in severity.

He taught that each person has a lifelong purpose that needs to be accomplished. The psyche has a need to grow and sometimes the individual takes what could be a wrong direction, and things occur that prevent the psyche from growing as it should. Depression occurs because the libido or psychic energy is sucked down into the unconscious. Effectively, the psyche has done this in order to shut down so that the person can reflect on the wrong direction. Treatment is not aimed at getting rid of the depression, but at helping the individual's psyche to understand and get back on track.

Alfred Adler and individual psychology

Adler believed that man's primary motivation was the will to gain power. He was the first person to coin the term 'inferiority complex', relating it to every child's experience that they are vulnerable and are surrounded by more powerful adults. As the person develops they will strive to overcome this early inferiority. When things do not go right there may be a reinforcing of the inferiority complex and increasing dissatisfaction with one's life.

Viktor Frankl and logotherapy

Frankl was a Holocaust survivor. In establishing his philosophy of logotherapy, which would become known as the third Viennese school of psychotherapy, he taught that we have choice as to how we view things and that it is important to see meaning in life. One must work against a tendency to be pessimistic and try to become an optimist. More and more research supports this view, in that optimists generally cope better with illness.

Frankl developed his theories while he was an inmate in the concentration camps and was able to use them to help many of his fellows who were depressed and suicidal.

One of the most important of Frankl's concepts was that of *anticipatory anxiety*. This is actually more than simply the fear that one has before an event. It is the anxiety about something happening, which actually is more likely to make it happen. For example, if you worry that you won't sleep then you probably will not.

Frankl believed that depression occurs at the psychological, physiological and spiritual levels. Psychologically, this results from feelings of inadequacy when trying to attempt things beyond your ability. Physiologically, the energy would leach away. And spiritually, it comes when there is tension about who you are in relation to who you think you should be.

The aim of logotherapy is to change the attitude towards how you feels about life and to remove that important anticipatory fear. In logotherapy. a technique of *paradoxical intention* is used instead.

Let us use the example of insomnia, which is of course so common in depression. People troubled with it usually go to bed and try too hard to sleep, the result being that they cannot sleep. With paradoxical intention you try to do the exact opposite. That is, you go to bed and you try 'not to sleep'. You may be amazed at how hard it then is to stay awake.

Another example is having an attack of hiccups. Instead of trying to stop them, try to make yourself hiccup. Offer yourself ten pounds to hiccup again. This paradoxical intention method usually makes them just stop.

Behaviourist psychology

This approach followed the work of Ivan Pavlov. Pavlov had done work on the 'conditioned reflex' and coined the term after his famous salivating dog experiments.

Pavlov was conducting experiments on digestion, including analysis of the contents of saliva and the conditions that caused saliva to be produced. To do this, he surgically implanted a cannula into the salivary glands of several dogs so that he could directly collect and measure their saliva. He observed that the dogs drooled not only when they were being fed, but also when no food was being given. It seemed that they were salivating when they saw his laboratory-coated assistants approach.

Pavlov aimed to understand why the appearance of the laboratory coats should have any bearing on the dogs' saliva production. The sight of a laboratory coat would not in itself seem a likely stimulus to salivation.

He therefore conducted a series of experiments in which the dogs were caged and then exposed to various stimuli, including using a buzzer when they were fed.

Pavlov concluded that the dogs had developed a response to the laboratory coats after all just as he was able to make them drool when a sound was made that they had associated with food. This new response became known as a conditioned response and, ultimately, the process that induced it was termed *classical conditioning.*

A conditioned reflex is the simplest form of learned behaviour. It is a new or modified response that arises from a process of conditioning, from a different, neutral stimulus rather than from the original stimulus with which it was paired.

The essence of behaviourist theory is that behaviours and emotions are learned. In the same way that one can learn to be fearful in certain situations, depression can also be learned. People who are depressed have learned helplessness, perhaps because they were overprotected when they were young. The pressure of life may seem too hard to cope with, and because they had learned from their parents to be passive, because they were always looked after, they feel unable to cope on their own and their self-worth and self-esteem diminish. The result is depression.

The behavioural approach utilises various psychological methods to help the individual alter their behaviour and thence improve the way they approach things and how they feel emotionally.

Cognitive behavioural psychology

This is a development from the behavioural model, developed by Aaron Beck. His view is that people with depression use or have learned to use a type of thinking that distorts reality.

When one is depressed there is a tendency to distort reality by utilising negative thinking about everything. People with depression tend to relate everything to themselves, be oversensitive and take everything personally, even when there is no reason to do so. They view the future as a dim prospect and they develop a lack of faith in their ability to perform in the future or to be able to deal with whatever the future holds. They may have high expectations of themselves that are unrealistic and they learn to expect themselves to fail.

Cognitive Behavioural Therapy looks at the dysfunctional emotions, maladaptive behaviours and cognitive processes that people experience and use and then, by using goal-oriented techniques, aims to get the person to alter the way that they think about the world, themselves and how they relate to other people. It also aims to help people to understand that their behaviours will affect their thoughts and their emotions. It can be extremely effective in treating depression.

Neuro-organic psychiatry – the biological theories

This subscribes to the view that mental activity is a product of brain function. Conditions like depression therefore may be the result of organic changes within the brain, or of imbalance in various neurotransmitters. These are caused by illnesses affecting brain function.

Support for these views has come from family studies which suggest that there is a possible genetic tendency. If a gene is turned on then depression becomes a possibility.

There have also been several theories about the biochemical nature of depression. The following have gained the most attention: Monoamine Hypothesis and Cytokine Hypothesis.

The Monoamine Hypothesis

In 1965, Dr Joseph Schildkraut published a paper entitled *The Catecholamine Hypothesis of Affective Disorders*.[4] He drew on the discoveries that the monoamine oxidase inhibitor drug isoniazid, which had been used for the treatment of tuberculosis, and the tricyclic drug imipramine, which had been developed as a substitute for the antipsychotic drug chlorpromazine, could actually elevate mood. Neither had been developed for treating depression, the effect was simply a chance discovery. On that basis, however, he postulated that deficiency of monoamine neurotransmitters, or natural messenger chemicals in the brain, had a significant role in depression. Hence it was called the Monoamine Hypothesis.

The Monoamine Hypothesis seems to account for the way in which most of the antidepressants that are commonly prescribed work.

It has its critics, however, since these antidepressants do not work for everyone who is depressed, and it does not seem to account for the fact that, although monoamine oxidase inhibitor drugs and tricyclic antidepressants (which we shall discuss in Chapter 7) elevate the levels of neurotransmitters within hours, a clinical effect does not take place for two weeks.

The Cytokine Hypothesis

Cytokines are small protein molecules found in the brain, central nervous system and the immune system. They are involved in cell-signalling, meaning that they transmit information between cells and may be involved in instructing them to carry out particular functions or actions.

High levels of cytokines are found in people with inflammatory conditions. They are also found in those suffering from depression, which has led researchers to think there may be a link between inflammation and depression. This is of quite marked importance, because it suggests, that for some people, depression is a symptom of an inflammatory process that is subtly affecting the brain.

An interesting study from Australia was published in the *Journal of Psychotherapy and Psychosomatics* in the autumn of 2010.[5] They selected a group of patients who had previously been selected for the Geelong Osteoporosis Study 1994–1997. There had been 1,494 women randomly recruited into the study. Of these, 837 were aged over 50 years. After ten years of follow-up, 386 agreed to take a psychiatric interview to determine whether any had become depressed.

The researchers were specifically interested in the use of statins and aspirin, but also collected information about other NSAIDs (non-steroidal anti-inflammatory drugs, like ibuprofen), paracetamol, hormones, antidepressants and drugs for diabetes. They performed a retrospective study of a control group with no history of depression, for the same period of time.

They found that 63 patients had a history of depression, but 41 were excluded because they had their depression diagnosed before the age of 50, which was one of the criteria used for inclusion into this study. This therefore gave them 22 cases to study.

Of the other women in the original group of 383, there were 323 who were eligible to be included as controls, since they had no depression.

Their findings were that:

- The prevalence or use of statins and aspirin was lower in the women who had a history of depression.

- Exposure to or use of statins was only 1 in 22 women with depression.

- Exposure to or use of statins was 93 in 323 women with no depression.

- Exposure to or use of aspirin (before the history of depression) was only 1 in 22 women with depression.

- Exposure to or use of aspirin was 103 in 323 women with no depression.

This led them to conclude that there was a highly significant reduction in the risk of developing major depression if one is taking aspirin or a statin. They could not explain the difference on the basis of lifestyle or of other drugs.

It seems that the reduction in inflammation seems to be the crux of the matter. This is entirely in keeping with the Cytokine Hypothesis and with the known facts about the ability of aspirin and statins to reduce inflammation.

The Cytokine Hypothesis has been submitted to a series of clinical trials around the world over the last few years and the evidence is really very compelling. Indeed, according to the Psychiatric Research into Inflammation, Immunity and Mood Effects (PRIME), a consortium of UK researchers, there is clear evidence that suggests that anti-inflammatory drugs like aspirin should be used alongside antidepressants in some cases. They may have a significant role to play in people with treatment-resistant depression, a chronic state in which people do not seem to respond to standard treatment. We will look at this in **Chapter 13, Treatment-resistant depression** and then again in **Chapter 15, A healthy diet**.

The Diathesis-Stress Theory of Depression

This theory suggests that depression may be caused by a combination of nature and nurture. Essentially, it considers that a genetic liability interacts with negative life experiences to cause depression. The word 'diathesis' derives from the Greek and indicates liability or vulnerability. If one has inherited a high liability then, according to this theory, it will not take a great deal of stress to tip you into depression. On the other hand, someone else with a low liability will require greater stressor experiences to make them depressed.

Thanks to advances in genetics it is possible to conduct research into this matter. Past studies have suggested that the neurotransmitter dopamine may have a role in depression. It is also known that rejection by one's parents is a risk factor for depression. A study led by Gerald Haeffel at the University of Notre Dame looked at this interaction by studying 177 male adolescents from a juvenile detention centre in Russia.[6] They used a structured interview to diagnose depression, coupled with a questionnaire that would assess various aspects of maternal parent rearing. They also were able to determine whether or not individuals had a gene associated with dopamine. They found that in those boys who had the gene and who had 'rejecting mothers', the risk of depression and suicidal thoughts was significantly higher than in those who had one factor or the other, or neither. It implies that neither nature nor nurture are enough on their own, but a combination of the two can cause depression.

A mixed bag

It should be fairly clear from reading through this chapter that there are several interesting theories, any one of which may explain why one is feeling depressed. Yet there may be more than one explanation in any case. What it comes down to is this, that there are a range of theories, each of which has had a treatment developed from it. They may be talking therapies, based upon the psychodynamic theories, or drug treatments based upon the concept that brain chemistry has been altered in some way. What we now need to look at is how all of these possible treatments could be mobilised to help someone who is depressed. This we shall do in Part Two.

PART TWO

DEALING WITH DEPRESSION

This part looks at the help that is available for people who feel depressed. It can be a bewildering journey for many people and a daunting prospect to actually take the first step. But no one should be intimidated and help *is* always available.

We shall also look at getting help for specific types of depression.

Chapter 5

Asking for help

It is not so much our friends' help that helps us, as the confidence of their help. Epicurus (341 BC–270 BC), philosopher and founder of the school of Epicureanism

Asking for help is often one of the hardest things that you can do when you are feeling depressed. For many people, to tell someone that they are not coping is akin to admitting defeat. This is a fallacy. It is not an admission of defeat, but an incredibly sensible and useful step to take towards treating depression. The problem with just soldiering on and suffering in silence is that often the suffering gets worse until the soldier loses all fight.

The fact is that, for many people who are starting to feel depressed, confiding in someone will often help enormously.

Epicurus and ancient Greek psychotherapy

Let me tell you a little about Epicurus, the philosopher who founded the school of Epicureanism. He was a scientist even before the concept of science had been developed. He taught that things should not just be believed, but should be tested. That is, he told his students that they should not blindly accept the teachings about the gods of Olympus, but should test everything through observation and logical deduction.

He also taught that happiness and pleasure resulted when there was an absence of suffering. His ideas were taken up by Asclepides of Bithynia, a Greek physician who would introduce these ideas to Rome. He actually treated his patients who suffered from mental distress of one form or another, many of whom would have been depressed, by talking and sharing their problems, by listening to music and by encouraging exercise and a good diet.

It was a good holistic approach that would work for many today.

KEY POINTS

You should seek help if:

- You are feeling sad and low in spirits and it is not getting any better, or if they are getting worse

- These feelings are affecting your work, your relationships and your life

- You start to have morbid thoughts about self-harming.

Friends and family

If you have a close relationship with a family member, then confide in them. Often the mere process of talking about how you feel will be enough to trigger some improvement and make you realise that people care about you. It may be that a parent or a brother or sister has felt something similar in the past and they are able to help you to understand it.

For some people, there may be reasons why they do not feel comfortable talking with family members about these deep feelings.

In that case, seek a friend, especially one who you know will be supportive.

Of course, some people feel that they do not have any close family or close friends in whom they can confide. If you feel this way, know that there are always people you can turn to: the Samaritans or your GP are always eager to help. However, this situation might be an indicator that you have been subconsciously isolating yourself from friends and family. This often happens to people when they get depressed, because they find that the interaction with others drains their energy. This creates a vicious cycle in that they get lonely and the lack of social interaction reinforces the mistaken belief that they are unlikeable and unworthy. Family and friends may be much more concerned than you think.

If anyone offers their time to have a chat, accept it.

Your GP

About 80 per cent of people who feel depressed do not seek treatment. The reasons for this are often to do with a feeling of embarrassment about being diagnosed with depression, as if it was something to be ashamed about. This is categorically not true. There is no reason to be ashamed of your feelings, especially if they are causing you difficulties.

Other people are concerned that a diagnosis of depression on their medical records could impair their chances of getting medical insurance or a mortgage. This is not the case. Depression is no different from having any physical condition. You would not feel embarrassed about having sciatica or chronic back pain, so why should you feel embarrassed about being depressed?

Some people hate the idea of having to take drugs, but drugs are not always necessary. Your GP will discuss how you are feeling and aim to see how he or she can best help you, personally. Gone are the days when 'doctor knows best' and a prescription was the outcome of every consultation. Nowadays, drug treatment will only be considered after it has been agreed between the patient and the doctor that this is the best course of action.

It may be that the GP will ask you to come back for further appointments to explore the situation further and to offer support during those sessions. Or it may be considered that you would benefit from being referred on to another person or agency.

Your health visitor

If you are a new mother you will have the support of your health visitor and you will be encouraged to talk about how you are feeling. Indeed, because of this and the importance of detecting postnatal depression new mothers are given the help they need at an early stage.

The health visitor is employed by the NHS and has a wide role in the early years of a family. They are fully trained nurses or midwives who have taken further advanced training in health visiting. A health visitor will stay involved and will provide support and advice until a child is aged five.

Counsellors

Many organisations, both educational and commercial, offer counselling to staff and students. There are different types of counselling and having a word with your line manager may be a good place to start. Your GP may also advise and arrange a course of counselling. We shall return to this in the next chapter.

Samaritans

Sometimes talking to someone who you do not know may seem a more acceptable option. In that case, contacting Samaritans may be worth considering.

Samaritans is a registered charity, founded in 1953 by the Reverend Chad Varah, a London vicar. He conceived it as an organisation that would help anyone who felt suicidal or emotionally distressed. It was very much an emergency organisation and it grew rapidly from one base until there are now over 200 branches across the UK and Ireland.

It now offers support to anyone in emotional distress. It is non-religious and it is apolitical. It is dependent on voluntary support, both financially and in terms of trained volunteers. Currently, there are over 20,000 trained volunteers who together provide a 24 hour, 365 days a year service. This is predominantly through telephone calls, but a confidential email service is also provided.

The aim of Samaritans is not to judge, provide advice or direct. It is to listen, ask questions and help the individual to explore their feelings in order to help them to see how they can best deal with their distress.

It is a misconception that you have to be suicidal in order to contact Samaritans. This is not the case. Over 80 per cent of people who contact them are not suicidal. So if you feel that you just need to talk to someone about how you feel, give them a call. The helpline number is in the Directory at the back of this book.

Chapter 6

How your doctor can help

The art of medicine is to cure sometimes, relieve often and comfort always.　　　　　Ambroise Paré (1510–1590), surgeon and physician

Think of your GP as your family friend and health advisor. That is, after all, the essence of good general practice. You can rest assured that at every consultation your doctor's aim is to arrive at the best way of helping whoever is occupying the patient's chair at that moment in time. Doctors are caring people, which is why they chose to enter medicine in the first place. So the first thing to do is go in and tell your doctor how you feel, and you can expect to be listened to, and helped.

Diagnosis

We talked about the range of symptoms that are commonly experienced in depression in Chapter 1. Well, from what you tell your doctor he or she will be trying to determine whether or not you are depressed and to arrive at a diagnosis.

The word diagnosis comes from the Greek *dia*, meaning 'through', and *gnosis*, meaning 'knowledge'. In essence it means 'find the answer through knowledge of the facts of the case'. It is not just a label that is arrived at, but a formulation of what the individual is suffering from and what has caused it.

Diagnosis is not always easy, because it is quite hard for both patient and doctor to be objective about subjective feelings. Your doctor may well use a standardised form such as the Patient Health Questionnaire.

The Patient Health Questionnaire (PHQ-9)

The PHQ-9 is a self-administered multiple-choice questionnaire, which was developed by Pfizer. It has been put in the public domain and can be accessed by the public from the Internet.

Essentially, it asks nine questions, each of which are considered criteria for making a diagnosis of depression. The individual scores them from 0, when the answer is 'never', to 3, when the answer is 'nearly every day'. A score out of 27 is obtained and the score gives an indication if depression is present and also its severity.

Doctors can also use this as a means to assess how someone is responding to treatment, when the score should progressively go down.

It has to be stated that this is not a fully diagnostic test, since it will not pick up on conditions that may not be depression, but which could still be of relevance. Yet it is a good indicator that anyone can do to assess whether they need help. If the reader takes this themselves and scores 5 or above then there would be very reasonable grounds to book an appointment to see your doctor to assess together where you go from there.

PATIENT HEALTH QUESTIONNAIRE (PHQ-9)	
Over the last 2 weeks, how often have you been bothered by any of the following problems?	
Little interest or pleasure in doing things?	Not at all Several days More than half the days Nearly every day
Feeling down, depressed, or hopeless?	Not at all Several days More than half the days Nearly every day
Trouble falling or staying asleep, or sleeping too much?	Not at all Several days More than half the days Nearly every day
Feeling tired or having little energy?	Not at all Several days More than half the days Nearly every day
Poor appetite or overeating?	Not at all Several days More than half the days Nearly every day
Feeling bad about yourself – or that you are a failure or have let yourself or your family down?	Not at all Several days More than half the days Nearly every day

Trouble concentrating on things, such as reading the newspaper or watching television?	Not at all Several days More than half the days Nearly every day
Moving or speaking so slowly that other people could have noticed? Or the opposite – being so fidgety or restless that you have been moving around a lot more than usual?	Not at all Several days More than half the days Nearly every day
Thoughts that you would be better off dead, or of hurting yourself in some way?	Not at all Several days More than half the days Nearly every day
Total = /27	
Depression Severity: 0–4 None, 5–9 mild, 10–14 moderate, 15–19 moderately severe, 20–27 severe.	

PHQ-9 is ©Pfizer. Reprinted with permission of Pfizer Limited.

The PHQ-9 has been validated by a study as being 88 per cent sensitive and specific for picking up major depression.[7, 8]

Other scales that your GP may use

The PHQ-9 is simple to use and in the time constraints of general practice it is probably the most widely used, since it takes a mere few minutes to do. Yet there are others that may be of even greater use, since they may assess things other than simply depression.

The Hospital Anxiety and Depression Scale (HAD) has also been tried out and found to have a validity in general practice. It takes about five minutes to do and it measures anxiety as well as depression. This can be very important if anxiety is a major component of how the individual is feeling. The anxiety and depression scales both have seven questions and a score will indicate normal, mild, moderate or severe.

The Beck Depression Inventory, Second Edition also takes about five minutes. It assesses depression as being minimal, mild, moderate or severe.

There are also others that may be used for children and adolescents and also for the elderly.

Mobilising help

The sort of help that your doctor may offer is likely to depend upon how severe the depression is, according to the score obtained on whichever scale has been used.

Mild depression

Doctor and patient may decide that the depression, assuming that has been diagnosed, can be managed by repeated attendances at the doctor's surgery. This is very reasonable for mild and even moderate depression.

You are also likely to be given advice on:

- *Self-help* – you may be given advice about exercise and lifestyle and possibly literature in the form of leaflets about depression, recommended self-help books and simple strategies that you can use.

- *Referral to local self-help groups* – there are many of these throughout the country and they welcome members. They are usually developed and coordinated by volunteers, who are called Group Facilitators. They do not aim to give individual advice and they are not experts in depression, but many people with depression find the network that they offer is of inestimable value.

- *Pen friends* – this is actually a scheme run by Depression Alliance. People with depression can be put in touch with a pen friend who has had experience of depression. This can be either a letter-writing pen friend or an email pen friend. For many people who are not comfortable with talking or being part of a group this may be very useful (see Directory).

- *Online CBT* (Cognitive Behavioural Therapy) may be advised.

ONLINE CBT – BEATING THE BLUES

The Department of Health recommend the use of this CBT online programme to help control mild-to-moderate depression: www.beatingtheblues.co.uk
It consists of a course of eight online sessions, each lasting an hour. No computer experience is needed.

Moderate depression

This severity of depression is likely to be having quite an impact on you, making work and possibly home life fairly difficult. Your GP may again be able to offer personal ongoing support in the surgery, but it is likely that you would be offered self-help as with mild depression, and probably also some form of talking therapy:

- Counselling – it may be decided and agreed that a course of talking therapy may be appropriate.

- Cognitive Behavioural Therapy (CBT), from a clinical psychologist.

- Some form of psychotherapy from either a psychiatrist or a professional member of the Community Mental Health Team who is suitably trained in psychotherapy, for example, a psychiatric nurse (we shall consider these in Chapter 8).

- Community Mental Health Team – if further help is needed with other professionals (see below).

- If a period off work would help then a wellness certificate may be given. This would likely be for a short period at first, but can be extended according to circumstances and the ongoing management of the condition.

Severe or major depression

With this order of severity there is more chance that the person could harbour or develop greater feelings of worthlessness and may be actively suicidal. The sort of treatments that are likely are:

- Antidepressants – there are a large number of such drugs, which the GP will probably initiate. We shall consider these in the next chapter.

- Combined treatment – it is quite likely that your doctor will recommend antidepressant medication together with a form of talking therapy. It is found that having antidepressants and CBT is more effective for people with moderate and severe depression than the use of one or the other on its own.

• Referral to the Community Mental Health Team.

KEY POINT

There is inevitable overlap between the three groups of mild, moderate and severe depression. In general, doctors aim at a holistic approach with depression and will tailor the management plan to suit the individual's needs.

The Community Mental Health Team

The way that mental health services are organised is in a constant state of change. At the moment, if further help is needed then the person may be referred to the Community Mental Health Team, or CMHT.

In most areas there are about 8–16 professionals in the team. They will have different training and different areas of expertise.

A referral by your doctor to the CMHT will result in a mental health worker, either a social worker or a psychiatric nurse or a psychologist, seeing you either individually or in a group. This could take place in the surgery if there is such an arrangement, or in a clinic or outpatient department.

The CMHT team includes:

Psychiatrist

This is usually a consultant psychiatrist although there may be associate specialists and psychiatrists in training who will assist. They are medically qualified, with postgraduate training in mental illness and emotional problems.

If the mental health worker considers that you need to see a psychiatrist, for example because they believe drug treatment is likely, then they will arrange an appointment.

You would undoubtedly benefit from the psychiatrist's expertise. During the consultation the psychiatrist will take an in-depth history that will look at how you feel and the events leading up to it. The discussion will be wide ranging and will give the psychiatrist a rounded picture of you and what you are experiencing. They will make a diagnosis and arrange a further follow-up either with themselves or with another member of the team. If antidepressant drugs are indicated they will prescribe them or liaise with the GP who will prescribe and monitor them.

Community psychiatric nurse (CPN)

As the title indicates, a CPN is a psychiatrically trained nurse who works in the community. They are often the key worker involved and will have experience of depression and its treatment. They will talk, lend a professional ear and advise. They will also monitor medication that has been prescribed. Some are also trained in psychotherapy.

Clinical psychologist

The psychologist is not a medically trained professional, but is someone who has a degree in psychology and who has taken a three-year postgraduate training in clinical psychology. Some have taken a doctorate and are entitled to use the title doctor, although this is not a medical degree.

They are experts in psychological treatments. They will often use problem-solving exercises, cognitive behavioural therapy and possibly other talking therapies.

Social worker

Many social workers specialise in mental health. They will be capable of talking with you about your troubles and may be of great practical use in helping to solve problems that might arise, for example with finance or housing.

Occupational therapist

This professional is trained in all things to do with the practical aspects of life (the 'occupational' refers to how you are occupied rather than what your occupation is). They look at and help assess what one is able to do and can advise about how to do practical things that will help. This may be to do with crafts, arts and activities that will help restore confidence and esteem.

Art therapist

Some CMHTs have trained artists who run art groups which help the individual to express themselves. Again, self-confidence and esteem may be helped considerably.

We shall return to this in Chapter 17.

Pharmacist

This professional is an expert in the preparation and delivery of drugs. They may have a special role in the treatment of depression and the types of drugs that may be appropriate for an individual. They would work with the psychiatrist who prescribes the drugs, the CPN who may monitor the drug, and the GP who is in charge of the ongoing care of the person.

Receptionists and secretaries

Very often, these professionals will be the friendly face that greets you when you arrive and register. Their input is more important than simply carrying out administrative duties, as their demeanour will be welcoming and should help to put you at ease before your appointments.

KEY POINTS

Your GP will make the first assessment as to whether you are depressed and whether you have mild, moderate or severe depression. According to this, you may be offered any combination of the following:

- Self-help strategies, including self-help group referral
- Referral for talking therapy
- Antidepressants drug prescription
- Referral to the CMHT and a psychiatrist.

Chapter 7

Medication for depression

It is much more important to know what sort of a patient has a disease than what sort of a disease the patient has.

Sir William Osler (1849–1919), physician

A couple of chance discoveries

The treatments for depression, or melancholia as it was called in the past, were always hit and miss. In his book, *The Anatomy of Melancholy*, Richard Burton described using self-help and music and sharing problems back in the seventeenth century. He also discussed various drugs that were then thought to have been of value. Many of them were probably little more than placebos.

In the modern era of medicine the first effective antidepressant drug was actually discovered by chance. It was noticed that when patients with tuberculosis received the drug Isoniazid, some actually experienced a lifting of their mood and were stimulated to greater activity. It was because of this that it was investigated and found to be a useful drug for treating depression. It was then marketed as Iproniazid. The first breakthrough had been made.

The second effective antidepressant drug was imipramine. This belongs to the group of drugs now called tricyclic antidepressants. It was developed from a drug called chlorpromazine, the first antipsychotic drug that had been synthesised in 1950. The aim was to try to produce a drug that had fewer side effects than chlorpromazine. Imipramine, a drug with three rings of atoms (hence the name 'tricyclics'), was initially thought to be a sedative. After a trial of the drug in 1955 by Dr Ronald Kuhn, a Swiss psychiatrist, it was found to have an antidepressant effect. However, it was found that in some patients it actually triggered episodes of mania.

These findings led Dr Joseph Schildkraut to publish his Monoamine Hypothesis (see Chapter 4).

THE PLACEBO EFFECT

A placebo is a drug or treatment which has no medical effect, but may still cause an improvement in the patient's condition if they believe it to be a real drug. The word comes from the Latin *placere*, meaning to please.

The 'placebo effect' is a fascinating phenomenon, possibly the most fascinating phenomenon in medicine. For some reason, an individual will respond to an inactive agent in a very positive manner. Nowadays, placebos are used in scientific trials, usually double-blind trials, in which neither the patient nor the doctor knows whether they are being given an active agent or a placebo. This sort of trial is used to assess whether a drug (the active agent) is superior to the placebo, i.e. better than nothing. The problem is that a placebo response can occur in anything between 25 and 70 per cent of cases. The frequently reported placebo response is 30 per cent, but it depends upon many factors. In general, the more dramatic the treatment, the greater the placebo response. It is also thought that the more the treatment is 'sold' by the enthusiasm of the practitioner, the greater will be the placebo effect.

Antidepressants

Today several types of antidepressants are available, which have been found to have fewer side effects than the two mentioned above.

We will now go through them group by group, in the order in which they were discovered.

KEY POINTS

- Most antidepressants do not start working for two to three weeks.

- After an antidepressant drug has been taken for eight or more weeks it should be discontinued slowly over four weeks, otherwise withdrawal effects are likely, e.g. nausea, headaches, worsening of symptoms and rebound effect, anxiety and restlessness.

- All antidepressant drugs can reduce sodium levels to produce 'hyponatraemia'. This can cause weakness, drowsiness, confusion and even convulsions. This is most common with the SSRIs.

- Antidepressants have been linked to suicidal thoughts, particularly in children and the young. They should be carefully monitored and if anyone develops such thoughts when on these drugs they should consult their doctor straight away.

- Antidepressant drugs may harm a developing foetus, so it is important not to become pregnant while taking them without first discussing the risks with your doctor.

GENERIC AS OPPOSED TO BRAND NAMES

The generic name of the drugs is supplied here. This is the actual name of the drug as opposed to the brand name. There may be several pharmaceutical companies who manufacture a drug and produce it under their brand names. The generic names are used by doctors to prescribe the drugs on the NHS prescription. For a list of brand names, see the *British National Formulary*, BNF.

Monoamine oxidase inhibitors (MAOIs)

This group of drugs paved the way in the pharmacological treatment of depression. They are not used very often today in the primary treatment of depression, because they interact with many foodstuffs and other drugs to produce unpleasant reactions. Yet they do still have a role, especially in people who fail to respond to tricyclic drugs or SSRI drugs (see below). They are thus second- or third-line drugs.

MAOI drugs may help people who seem to have:

- Treatment-resistant depression – when there may actually be a dramatic response to a MAOI
- Severe phobias with depression
- Atypical depression
- Hypochondriacal symptoms and depression
- Hysterical symptoms and depression.

The MAOI drugs work by inhibiting an enzyme called monoamine oxidase. This results in an increase in amine neurotransmitters. Side effects come about because they also inhibit the metabolism by the body of various amine-containing drugs, called *sympathomimetics*, which are present in over-the-counter remedies like cough medicines. These can then have a 'pressor' effect on the body, which means that they can cause the blood pressure to rise dramatically. Warning symptoms of this are flushes and throbbing headaches.

Various foods that are rich in tyramine – cheese, pickles, broad beans and sandwich spreads or extracts like Oxo, Bovril and Marmite – may also have a pressor effect and produce a similarly dangerous effect if a MAOI drug is taken.

The problem with the earlier MAOI drugs was the fact that they are irreversible in their action. This meant that they permanently blocked the enzyme monoamine oxidase and it would take two weeks before the body could build up more of it. Therefore, a side effect affects the person for an unacceptably long time.

When taking a MAOI drug, great care should be taken to ensure that all food is fresh, not processed, and any food which could be less than fresh, such as game, fish or poultry, should be avoided.

Some patients who have a problem with their liver, whether or not through alcohol, can develop liver toxicity with these drugs.

The most commonly used drugs in this category are phenelzine and isocarboxazid.

Reversible MAOI

The MAOI drug moclobemide is indicated for major depression and social anxiety disorder. It is said to act by reversible inhibition of monoamine oxidase type A. More correctly, it should be termed a RIMA (reversible inhibitor of monoamine oxidase). It is considered a second-line drug.

MAOI antidepressants can interact with other drugs, so you should always ensure that your doctor is aware of any other drugs being taken.

KEY POINT

People prescribed MAOI drugs should take care to avoid over-the-counter preparations containing sympathomimetics and should avoid processed foods and cheese.

Tricyclic antidepressants (TCAs)

These are among the oldest drugs to be used in treating depression, but remain among the most commonly used, together with the SSRI drugs that we shall come to soon.

They are considered safer than the MAOIs, yet they still have to be used with caution with patients who have various other medical conditions:

Heart problems – because they have the potential to speed the heart up and cause abnormal heart rhythms.

Hyperthyroidism (an overactive thyroid gland) – because they can speed up the heart.

phaeochromocytoma (a tumour of the adrenal gland which produces excess adrenaline and noradrenaline) – because it could speed up the heart.

Glaucoma – raised pressure within the eye, which could be increased dramatically.

Prostate problems – retention of urine could be caused in men with prostatic hypertrophy.

Patients with a history of mania – which could be provoked by a TCA.

Constipation – can be worsened by TCA drugs.

It also needs to be used with caution when treating elderly patients. There is an increased chance that they may have several co-existent pathological conditions and may not metabolise drugs as well as younger people, so are more at risk of developing side effects. The tricyclic antidepressants need to be used in smaller doses to begin with and they need close monitoring to check the development of any side effects.

Having said this, when prescribed under the right circumstances they can be extremely effective and many doctors still consider them their first-line treatment for moderate depression.

Common side effects:

- Arrhythmias – irregular heart rhythms may be induced
- Postural hypotension – the blood pressure may drop causing faintness on getting up quickly
- Anxiety
- Dizziness
- Sleep disturbances
- Convulsions
- Hallucinations – seeing or hearing things that are not there
- Delusions – developing false beliefs that cannot be reasoned away
- Dry mouth
- Constipation
- Breast enlargement
- Sexual dysfunction
- Increased appetite and weight gain
- Liver and blood anomalies
- Nausea and vomiting
- Tinnitus
- Skin rashes
- Hair loss.

If side effects occur, the individual should always consult their doctor rather than suddenly stop taking the medicine, as the doctor may want to gradually reduce the dose rather than risk a rebound effect.

Tricyclic antidepressants can interact with other drugs, so you should always make your doctor aware of any other drugs being taken.

Common tricyclic antidepressant drugs used are amitriptyline, clomipramine, dosulepin, imipramine, nortriptyline and trimipramine.

Tricyclic-related antidepressants

These are newer drugs that are similar in effect to the tricyclics, yet have a different chemical make-up. The same side effects and cautions apply to them but, in addition, mianserin can cause blood anomalies and can affect the immune system. For that reason a full blood count should be taken every four weeks for three months and, if indicated, the drug should be discontinued. The doctor should also be consulted if an infection, sore throat or fever develop while taking the drug.

Commonly used drugs in this group are mianserin and trazodone.

Selective serotonin re-uptake inhibitors (SSRIs)

These are the newest and are generally considered the safest drugs for depression. Nowadays, they tend to be the first-line treatment when drugs are indicated.

They work by affecting chemical messengers called neurotransmitters which the brain cells use to communicate with each other. The SSRIs selectively affect serotonin instead of other neurotransmitters. They block the reabsorption – i.e. the *re-uptake* – of serotonin in the brain. This seems to help the brain cells to communicate with each other and lifts your mood.

SEROTONIN, THE HAPPINESS HORMONE

Serotonin is one of the main neurotransmitters in the body. Its proper name is 5-hydroxytryptamine or 5-HT. It is a monoamine neurotransmitter, which is mainly built up from the amino acid tryptophan. We shall return to this when we look at diet and depression in Chapter 15.

Only 20 per cent of the serotonin in the body is found in the brain and nervous system. The majority is found in certain cells in the gut, where its function is to regulate the way that the bowel moves.

People who are depressed may have lower levels in the brain, or the reabsorption or re-uptake drops the levels too much. The SSRIs may keep the levels topped up, so that brain cells function better and communicate with each other and the mood is lifted.

Commonly used SSRIs are citalopram, escitalopram, fluoxetine, fluvoxamine, paroxetine and sertraline.

Withdrawal reactions can occur with SSRIs. The risk of this is greatest with paroxetine. Such actions include:

- Gastro-intestinal reactions – diarrhoea, abdominal pains

- Headache

- Anxiety dizziness

- Pins and needles

- Fatigue

- Flu-like symptoms

- Palpitations

- Visual disturbances.

SSRI antidepressants can interact with other drugs and supplements so, as with all of these drugs, you should always make your doctor aware of any other drugs being taken.

SEROTONIN SYNDROME

Very rarely, a SSRI drug can cause serotonin levels to rise to a dangerous level. This can cause confusion, rapid heart rate, dilated pupils, fever and possibly loss of consciousness. It is a medical emergency and medical aid should be sought urgently.

It most usually occurs when, in addition to taking a SSRI drug, someone is taking another drug that boosts serotonin, St John's wort (a herbal preparation) or ginseng. Also, if too much of any of these other drugs is taken it can cause serotonin syndrome on its own:

- MAOIs
- Tricyclics
- Opiates – e.g. pethidine, entazocine, buprenorphine
- CNS stimulants – amphetamines, cocaine
- Triptans – used for migraine treatment
- Antihistamines – chlorpheniramine
- Anti-nausea drugs – e.g. metoclopramide
- Antipsychotics – e.g. olanzapine, risperidone
- Herbs – e.g. St John's wort, ginseng, nutmeg.

Other antidepressant drugs

These drugs affect other neurotransmitters and all tend to be reserved for the treatment of major depression.

Venlafaxine

This is a serotonin and noradrenaline re-uptake inhibitor (SNRI). It is less sedative and produces fewer side effects than the tricyclics. It can produce heartbeat irregularities, however, so it should still be used with caution. It has to be taken under supervision and should not be suddenly stopped, since it has a marked withdrawal effect.

It is always recommended that patients should have an electrocardiogram (ECG) before having it prescribed.

Mirtazepine

This is a pre-synaptic alpha2-adrenoceptor antagonist. That is a bit of a mouthful, but essentially it increases the transmission of impulses between nerve cells. It has sedative effects, but otherwise generally has few side effects.

Aglomelatine

This is a melatonin receptor agonist and a selective serotonin receptor antagonist. It is reserved for major depression.

Reboxitine

This is a selective inhibitor of noradrenaline reuptake. It is used for major depression.

Flupenthixol

This is a drug used in treating major depression and psychotic illness.

Duloxetine

This is a drug that inhibits the re-uptake of both serotonin and noradrenaline. It is used in treating major depression.

Tryptophan

This is an amino acid, so is found in foods; we shall look at this further in Chapter 15. It is actually licensed as an adjunct treatment for depression, when prescribed under supervision. Its place is seen to be in treatment-resistant depression.

Care should be taken, since it can produce a potentially dangerous neurological condition called eosinophilia-myalgia syndrome, or EMS.

EMS

This is a rare condition that was first described in 1989 after three cases were reported in New Mexico. It is an association of an *eosinophilia* (rise in the level of eosinophils, a particular type of white cell in the blood, often associated with allergic reactions) and marked myalgia, or muscle pains. An epidemic followed, affecting 1,500 people. Unfortunately, three people died. All of the cases had taken the supplement L-tryptophan.

The condition often improves after stopping the L-tryptophan, but not always, and debilitating symptoms can persist.

For this reason, L-tryptophan is not available in the UK as a supplement. It should only be prescribed by a specialist, and if any flu-like symptoms develop it should be stopped and investigations performed.

Anxiolytics

Drugs that reduce the symptoms of anxiety are sometimes used in the acute phase of depression, because in addition to the depressed mood the person may feel anxious, fearful, irritable and suffer from insomnia. These are the drugs that used to be called *tranquillisers*.

The SSRI drugs often are quite effective in reducing the anxiety as well as the depression, but sometimes they need to be supplemented by an anxiolytic or a hypnotic. An anxiolytic is a drug that reduces anxiety and a hypnotic is a drug that helps to induce sleep.

Benzodiazepines

The benzodiazepine group of drugs contains drugs that are both anxiolytic and hypnotic. Neither should be prescribed for long, since they very rapidly induce dependency. They are generally only seen as having a very short-term usage. The lowest dose possible should be prescribed and it should be stopped as soon as possible.

- Diazepam, oxazepam, lorazepam, chlordiazepoxide and alprazolam are all very effective anxiolytic drugs that relieve the symptoms of acute anxiety. They are prescription-only drugs, but few doctors will be willing to prescribe them for more than a few days.

- Nitrazepam, flurazepam, laprazolam, lormetazepam, and temazepam are all hypnotic or sleeping pills. They should only be used for very short periods.

The Z-drugs

This is the name given to a group of drugs that are not benzodiazepines, but act on the same receptors in the nervous system as do the benzodiazepines. These include zopiclone, zolpidem and zaleplon.

They are relatively short-acting and they tend to be prescribed for a short period. The National Institute for Health and Care Excellence (NICE) recommends that they should only be used for 2–4 weeks and then be discontinued.

Beta-blockers

These are drugs that are widely used in medicine because they are effective in lowering blood pressure. They also are quite effective in reducing the physical symptoms of anxiety, so they act as a physiological tranquilliser. They do not cause dependency problems, but some of them do cause side effects, so they should be used with caution in people with asthma and with low blood pressure. They may also cause sleep difficulties.

Other drugs

As we discussed earlier, some cases of depression may be caused by other conditions, or as a reaction to having a condition.

Hypothyroidism is associated with depression and therefore treatment of the underlying condition may improve depression. It is not that the drug used, L-thyroxine, has any antidepressant effect itself; rather that as the condition improves the depression lifts.

The same can occur in any chronic condition that significantly impacts upon one's life. Arthritis, heart conditions and strokes are all noted examples of this. Having said that, it may be that if the Cytokine Hypothesis is correct, the inflammation that is present in some conditions may directly cause depression by virtue of the rise in cytokines. Any drug that reduces that inflammation may therefore be treating both conditions at the same time.

Mood stabilisers

These are drugs used to control elevated mood and mania.

Lithium

This is the mainstay of treatment in manic states. It has been in use for 40 years, but amazingly, we still have no clear idea of how it works. It seems to have an effect on the way that messages are sent in the brain. It is used both in treatment and to maintain control of the mood.

It is important to have an ECG and regular blood tests before starting to take this medication to make sure that the level of lithium does not rise too high, since it can affect kidney and thyroid gland function.

Lithium side effects include:

- Dry mouth

- Metallic taste in the mouth

- Shakiness or slight trembling

- Looseness of the bowels

- Weight gain

- Fluid retention

- Thyroid gland underactivity.

Valproate

This is used as an alternative to lithium. It is an anticonvulsant or anti-epileptic drug. It seems to work as well as lithium, but may be slightly better at controlling rapid swings in mood. Sometimes it is used in combination with lithium.

Carbamazepine

This is an anti-epileptic drug that is also useful for neuralgia. It was the first of the anticonvulsant drugs found to be a mood-stabiliser. It can cause more side effects than valproate.

Lamotrigine

This is another anticonvulsant that is found to have mood-stabilising features. It is effective in controlling very low mood. It is not as effective with manic episodes. It has to have the dose increased slowly over several weeks, since it can cause a lot of skin problems.

Antipsychotics

This group of drugs is used in severe types of mental distress:

- Severe anxiety
- Severe depression
- Schizophrenia
- Bipolar disorder
- Postpartum psychosis.

These drugs used to be known as the Major Tranquillisers, although they are not actually tranquillising in their action. They have no relationship to the anxiolytics mentioned earlier. They are valuable in conditions where people feel detached from reality and they work to reduce and stop hallucinations and delusions. They work by affecting the neurotransmitters in the brain, especially dopamine.

There are two types:

Older antipsychotics

These are the first-generation drugs and are sometimes referred to as the 'typical' antipsychotics. They are strong in their action, but have quite marked side effects, including stiffness, trembling and reduction of libido. Examples are chlorpromazine, haloperidol, trifluoperazine and sulpiride.

Newer antipsychotics

These are the second-generation antipsychotics that have been developed in the last decade. They are also described as the 'atypical' antipsychotics. They also act on dopamine to block its action, but not as much as the older drugs. Consequently, they have fewer side effects affecting movement, but they do tend to provoke weight gain and their effect on libido and sexual function may be more profound. Examples are amisulpride, olanzapine, risperidone and zotepine.

St John's wort

This is a herbal remedy that is available to buy over the counter to treat mild depression. It is derived from the plant *Hypericum perforatum*, and is also known as Holy Herb, or Balm to the Warrior's Wound. It has traditionally been used for all sorts of stitch-like pains, toothache and neuralgia. It was used by Hippocrates as a wound healer and also as a treatment for melancholia.

It is interesting because it is a good example of the Doctrine of Signatures, the medieval belief that plants had a 'signature' that alerted man to their healing potential. The curiously perforated leaves were thought to represent the arrows that martyred St John. The plant blossomed around the saint's day, and the juice of the leaves, which is red, was thought to be like the blood of the saint.

It has been shown to be effective as an antidepressant in mild depression. It is, however, very important to talk with your doctor if you are considering taking St John's wort, since it can react with several orthodox medicines, including:

- Antidepressants – it can cause the serotonin syndrome (see p. 88)
- Anticonvulsants
- Anti-HIV drugs
- Cyclosporin
- Digoxin
- Warfarin
- Oral contraceptives
- Theophylline.

Chapter 8

Talking therapies

Thinking: the talking of the soul with itself.

Plato (427–347 BC), Greek philosopher

Psychotherapy is the collective name given to the various types of talking therapy. Sometimes the simple process of talking about how you are feeling will help alleviate symptoms. Some people find that talking in a group suits them and that it is helpful to talk with other people who feel similarly. Just knowing that you are not alone with your feelings can be therapeutic. On the other hand, others may feel threatened or uncomfortable with the idea of talking about themselves in front of a number of strangers. They may benefit more from an individual approach with a single therapist. There are pros and cons with both approaches and you can discuss this with your doctor or the therapist that you are referred to in the Community Mental Health Team.

Who offers talking therapies?

There is an array of people who practise talking therapies. Not all talking therapists are doctors, however.

Let's look at who might offer psychotherapy.

Psychiatrist – a medical doctor trained in the diagnosis and treatment of mental illness. They can prescribe drugs. Some psychiatrists may take additional training in psychotherapy.

Clinical psychologist – they are not medically trained and cannot prescribe drugs. They have taken postgraduate training in talking therapies. They may offer CBT.

Nurse psychotherapists – they are qualified nurses who have taken postgraduate training in psychotherapy.

UKCP member psychotherapists – they are usually graduates who have undergone postgraduate training exclusively in psychotherapy. If they are registered with the UK Council for Psychotherapy (UKCP), they will have undertaken four years of postgraduate training.

UKCP member psychotherapeutic counsellors – they have taken a UK Council for Psychotherapy (UKCP), course in therapeutic counselling and are recognised as competent counsellors.

Counsellors – these are therapists who hold a qualification in counselling, such as those accredited by the British Association of Counselling and Psychotherapy (BACP), or another organisation.

Something to be aware of

While one can see that antidepressant drugs may have side effects, you may not think that talking therapies could have any problems.

They are generally very safe, but because talking about your feelings and experiences may bring memories to the surface they can be uncomfortable for a while.

In addition, if the talking involves examining relationships the person is involved in, this may cause some stress in the relationships as the person questions and examines the nature of those relationships. It can cause family tension, for example.

All in all, the main thing is to have trust in the therapist that you are seeing. A good starting point is to ensure that they are qualified and experienced. No therapist should be evasive or appear offended by your questions, because if they are adequately trained they should expect this and be happy to reassure you. Do not think that you will hurt their feelings by asking.

Improving Access to Psychological Therapies Programme (IAPT)

In the UK, it has long been recognised that many people with anxiety or depression would benefit from some form of talking therapy, the problem being that services were not always available locally. Even when they were, there could be a considerable waiting time. Indeed, a recent survey by the Mental Health Foundation found that 75 per cent of GPs had prescribed antidepressant medication when they felt that talking therapy would be more appropriate. The problem was in gaining access to talking therapies for their patients.

In 2007, the government responded to the National Institute for Health and Clinical Excellence (NICE) guidelines and injected a considerable amount of money into the Improving Access to Psychological Therapies Programme (IAPT). The aim is to make frontline psychotherapy services for both anxiety and depression available on the National Health Service (NHS). This could be used alongside drug treatment if deemed appropriate.

Initially, the programme targeted people of working age, but up until 2015 it is being gradually extended to provide talking therapies to all adults, children and young adults, and people with long-term health problems, medically unexplained symptoms and severe mental illness.

So far, the programme has been remarkably successful. By 2011, over 90 per cent of the Primary Care Trusts had access to psychotherapy services and over 3,500 cognitive behavioural therapists had been trained. These treatments were all free on the NHS.

NICE-approved talking therapies available on the NHS

The following talking therapies are approved by NICE and have a good evidence base for effectiveness in treating mild-to-moderate depression. That means that they are as effective in helping depression as anti-hypertensive drugs are in treating high blood pressure, influenza vaccination is in preventing flu, or surgery is in repairing hernias or removing cataracts:

- Counselling

- Cognitive Behavioural Therapy (CBT)

- Interpersonal Psychotherapy (ITP)

- Dynamic Interpersonal Therapy (DITP)

- Couple Therapy for Depression.

In addition, CBT and ITP are also both approved by NICE for the treatment of moderate-to-severe depression.

> ### KEY POINTS
>
> - You can expect your consultations to be confidential and that any information given to your therapist will only be shared with your GP or other professionals involved in your care.
> - Your progress will probably be self-assessed, usually by questionnaires and scoring after each session. This helps to monitor how you are responding to treatment, and makes sure that the treatment course is on the right track. If it appears not to be helping then the management plan can be readdressed.

Counselling

This is the simplest type of talking therapy. It may well be available in-house at your GP's surgery. Generally, a course of 6–10 sessions, each lasting 50–60 minutes will be arranged, usually at weekly or fortnightly intervals, according to how you can fit them into your schedule, over about 12 weeks.

The British Psychological Society defines counselling as a system intended to 'help people improve their sense of wellbeing, alleviate their distress, resolve their crises and increase their ability to solve problems and make decisions for themselves'.

An individual qualified counsellor will be assigned to you, so that you have continuity and can build up a rapport. The treatment that you receive will be tailored to your needs.

Often people with mild depression will respond well to just talking about their problems, the counsellor facilitating them in seeing how their problems are affecting them. In this way the problems may seem clearer, and because of this they may find ways of solving the problem. For example, it may help to come to terms with a life event.

From this point of view, counselling is not as complex as other talking therapies, which may aim to change the way that you think in general. Rather than doing this they will be focusing on how the person's feelings affect them and building a picture of things from their point of view. You can expect your counsellor to be empathic with you, but they will not offer advice on what you should do. They will help you to see things in different and more positive ways, rather than in a way that undercuts your self-esteem and self-worth.

Cognitive Behavioural Therapy (CBT)

'Cognitive' refers to thought and thinking, and 'behavioural' refers to the actions we take and the things that we do, so CBT is about looking at the way you think and how your thoughts affect the way you feel and the way you act.

CBT looks at the way that the individual has become depressed and the beliefs and patterns of negative thinking that they have developed which has locked them into their depressed mood. By the individual altering their thought pattern and developing positive outlooks and positive thinking, the depression often resolves itself.

CBT has been widely researched and is approved for the treatment of a wide range of conditions:

- Mild to severe depression
- Panic attacks
- General anxiety
- Phobias
- Anger management

- Habit disorders
- Chronic fatigue.

A course of CBT will generally involve 16–20 sessions over 3–4 months with a trained therapist, often a qualified clinical psychologist. In these sessions the focus will be on the present and the way that the person is thinking and feeling. A different way of thinking is developed and a plan made to test it out between then and the next session. The person is encouraged to write down their thoughts and their feelings as well, so that they can discuss them with their therapist. This is all very active and the person is very involved in their own treatment, since it must be the sufferer who alters the way that they think.

Group CBT

This is sometimes recommended. This will consist of a group of people who have similar feelings, meeting weekly, with two professional therapists leading the group.

Self-help CBT

This may actually be advised by your GP. There are programmes on the Internet which can be accessed by the individual, or self-help books that may be used effectively as 'low level' CBT, to deal with mild depression.

Mindfulness-Based Cognitive Therapy (MBCT)

This is an interesting therapy that has been developed over the last few years. It is showing excellent results in reducing the relapse rates in depression by up to 50 per cent. It is used between episodes to treat people who suffer from depression, to reduce or prevent relapses of depression.

It is a development from Mindfulness-Based Stress Reduction, which itself was based on Buddhist meditation techniques, that had been developed by John Kabat-Zinn.

MBCT is based on the concept of mindfulness, which means paying attention to the present moment, deliberately, without judgement. It is a means of experiencing the moment without being sucked into worrying how it is affecting you or your future.

It was developed by Zindel Segal and Mark Williams and is given in a course to groups of people with a past history of depression. A course last eight weeks, with a two-hourly instruction every week, then one day-long session per week from week five to seven. The individual is taught guided meditation and attempts to cultivate mindfulness in their practice throughout the week, and in their daily life. It is taught by an MBCT teacher.

MBCT has been endorsed by NICE as an effective prevention of depressive illness. It seems most effective in helping people who have experienced at least two episodes of depression.

It may be possible that it is available on the NHS in some localities, but if not then information may be available from the Oxford Mindfulness Centre:

MBCT, Prince of Wales International Centre
University of Oxford Department of Psychiatry
Warneford Hospital
Oxford OX3 7JX
Telephone/Voicemail: +44 (0)1865 613141
http://mbct.co.uk

Interpersonal Psychotherapy (ITP)

This is a talking therapy that aims to treat the type of depression that has arisen from your relationships with family and friends. If a problem has arisen it can affect your self-esteem, which can then make you withdraw or even isolate yourself from friends and family, who may in turn withdraw from you. This can make you feel that you are not worthy, which can lead to depression. It can be seen as both a cause and a consequence.

ITP is based on the idea that if you can improve the way you communicate and relate to others, you affect your emotions, which will often alleviate the symptoms of depression. It seems to be a good treatment for people with dysthymia.

By working to look at how the way you feel is affecting your relationships, and how your relationships are affected by your feelings, you may be able to resolve conflicts, change your perspective, develop better coping strategies and feel better.

ITP will often focus on things that may have triggered a depression:

- Life events

- Grief

- Broken relationships

- Conflict with others

- Problems and reasons why relationships cannot be maintained.

ITP can be used both for acute and maintenance therapy. That is, a course of around eight sessions may be given for a single episode of depression, over 8–12 weeks, but it is also possible that it can be used to maintain treatment at more widely spaced intervals over a longer time.

Dynamic Interpersonal Therapy (DIT)

This talking therapy may sound as if it is just a more high-powered version of ITP, but it is not as simple as that. 'Dynamic' means that it is a psychodynamic therapy. In this context, 'psychodynamic' means that it digs deep to bring true feelings to the surface, in other words it can stir up many thoughts and emotions. It is considered to be very useful for people who are depressed and who have relationship problems. They may have past relationship problems that they cannot get over and which affect their ability to form a relationship. This is seen to lead to distortions in the way that the person thinks and feels.

DIP is typically used over 16 sessions of 50–60 minutes each. During this time you will work on building a relationship with the therapist.

A set strategy is used consisting of three phases. There is an engagement/assessment phase, extending over the first four sessions, then a middle phase between sessions 5 and 12, and an ending phase over sessions 13 to 16. The therapist will work to a strategy with the client during each phase.

The therapist aims to use this relationship as a mirror to explore the pattern of other relationships you have had. For example, fears of rejection or of dependency in relationships in general may be explored and new ways of thinking can be developed and tested.

Couple therapy and family therapy

It may not be just the person who is depressed who has the problem, but it can be a result or a reflection of the dynamics within a couple or within a family. Accordingly, couple or family therapy may help.

- Both members of the couple would be invited, or all members of the family.
- The relationships would be looked at and explored.
- The way that everyone in the group thinks and feels would be explored.

The aim is not to give advice or guidance, but to allow couples or families to talk in a neutral environment with the therapist as a facilitator to understanding. It is non-judgemental, but usually immensely helpful.

One therapist or a pair of therapists may be present and the session may be recorded so that it can be played back at a later stage, either to other therapists who may be involved, or to other members of the family, or just to show the participants how they were reacting at various points. It facilitates communication and may help each person to understand their partner or the other members of the family.

This sort of therapy may need to go on for up to 20 sessions over six months. (See Relate in Directory.)

Other talking therapies

We have already considered the talking therapies that are approved by NICE, and which are available on the NHS. There are many other types of talking therapy or psychotherapy that may be available in the private sector. The fact that they are not approved by NICE does not mean that they are not effective.

Psychoanalysis

This is the popular image of psychotherapy, based on the theories of Sigmund Freud. This is a therapy that would need to be obtained privately. It involves a long period of analysis, over many months and even years.

The theory is that unacceptable thoughts develop in childhood and become repressed into the unconscious mind where they fester away to affect the emotions, thoughts and behaviour.

The patient or 'analysand' verbalises their thoughts and the psychoanalyst interprets the symbology of them in order to help the patient develop insight into the issues and problems that have been caused in the person's life.

In Freudian psychoanalytic terms, depression comes about through objective 'loss' of something that you had identified with. The unconscious construes these losses as a reason to blame yourself, so you feel unworthy and inferior as a result.

Jungian analysis

This is a type of psychotherapy based on the works of Carl Jung. The aim of therapy in this case is to expand the individual's consciousness to achieve balance and a sense of wellbeing.

The therapy sessions are regarded as very important and they occur very frequently, perhaps one or more times a week. Sessions will focus on patterns in life and difficulties experienced, in order that you can develop a sense of self-awareness, as the depression may have occurred as a sort of defence mechanism; a 'blowing of a fuse' that prevents further damage.

Jungian treatment aims to accept the state of 'being' and to look at what is going wrong in life. Like psychoanalysis, it is a lengthy process and requires commitment.

Logotherapy

This is a type of psychotherapy developed by Viktor Frankl, a Holocaust survivor. He survived and helped many of his fellow prisoners by persuading them that there is always meaning in life.

The essence of logotherapy, from the Greek *logos*, which translates as 'meaning', is to find meaning or purpose in life. There are three basic principles:

1. Life has meaning in every circumstance, even in suffering.

2. Our main motivation is our will to find meaning in life.

3. We have freedom to find meaning in what we do, and in what we experience.

It can be seen that it is an existential form of psychotherapy. It seems to work well with adolescents. Frankl believed that if people have goals that are unreachable, perhaps goals that have been placed upon them by powerful figures like their parents, then they experience a loss of the sense of their future, which makes them lose the sense of meaning in their life, which can result in depression. The aim of therapy is to change the attitude and to see meaning by creating achievable goals and to reassert meaningfulness and purpose.

Psychodynamic psychotherapy

Again, this is an analytic therapy that aims at bringing deep unconscious feelings to the surface where they can be examined and analysed. It looks at past experiences in order to see how they may have a bearing on current thinking and behaviour. This will include childhood and adolescent experiences and feelings. The therapist 'observes' and analyses the way that the patient or client projects or transfers feelings onto the therapist, all the while observing and interpreting the dynamics that are involved. For example, the person may transfer onto the therapist the feelings that they had about a parent.

KEY POINTS

A lot of analytical therapies, such as psychoanalysis and Jungian analysis, may stir things up in the short term, as unconscious memories and emotions are brought to the surface. This is more likely than with other talking therapies, such as counselling.

It is important to know that the therapist is adequately trained.

Group analysis

Some people respond well to group analysis. Part of the way this works is by enabling you to explore the way you function and relate to other people within a social group. If you can view the group as a mini-society, then by integrating and communicating with others it can produce lasting benefit in the way you feel about yourself and your place in their society.

The group leader or leaders facilitate, but do not actively participate. It is often a very successful means of helping people with mild-to-moderate depression.

Other psychotherapies

Art therapy, dance therapy and drama therapy use creativity as a means of exploring personal problems and emotions. We shall look at them in the last chapter of the book.

Transactional analysis

This is an interesting psychotherapy developed by Dr Eric Berne in the 1950s. It is based on the concept that the self has three components – the child, the adult and the parent. These parts communicate and form transactions in various situations, in which one will predominate. In transactional analysis (TA) the client can choose which role to adopt in a transaction, to modify behaviour. It also looks at the inner child and examines what needs were or were not met.

Neuro Linguistic Programming (NLP)

Neuro Linguistic Programming is a holistic technique that was developed by Richard Bandler and John Grinder in the 1970s. Their groundbreaking book *Frogs into Princes* was a bestseller and began an extremely useful therapeutic process that is widely used today.

The aim of NLP is to help you learn and create good and successful experiences, by looking at the way you think (neuro), how you communicate (linguistic), and how you can teach (programming) the mind to think, communicate and perform more successfully.

In NLP terms, depression comes about through having developed negative thought patterns and actions or behaviours and habits that undermine and sabotage your ability to feel happy. A NLP practitioner will help eliminate these negative thoughts and to develop behaviour that will not sabotage yourself, but help you to fulfil yourself and your potential.

There are three main techniques whereby a NLP practitioner will 'rewire' thinking processes to induce a positive frame of mind:

- Anchoring – the transfer of positive responses from one set of events or circumstances to another.
- Reframing – giving a different set of references or perspectives to create a positive world view.
- Teaching how to use metaphor – these are powerful ways to communicate with the unconscious. Jokes, stories, analogies and all manner of metaphors can open the unconscious mind to uncover hidden issues and aid them to be resolved.

Hypnotherapy

Hypnosis was first called Mesmerism after Dr Franz Anton Mesmer (1734–1815). Mesmer went to university in Vienna to study divinity, philosophy and law, but changed course and took up the study of medicine. He graduated in 1766, his doctoral thesis being entitled *De influxu planetarum in corpus humanum* – 'The Influence of the Planets upon the Human Body'.

In this he postulated that the whole universe was filled with a magnetic fluid and that the planets exerted an influence upon the human body through their effect on this invisible fluid. He believed that this energy could be harnessed by gifted individuals like himself to correct imbalances in patients. He called this phenomenon 'animal magnetism'.

The name 'hypnosis' was coined in 1841 by Dr James Braid, a Scottish surgeon, from the Greek *hypnos,* meaning sleep. He recognised that it was a form of sleep or trance-like state in which the individual became more suggestible.

Hypnotherapy is the application of the trance-like state for therapeutic purposes. In the trance state the individual is more suggestible and less critical of statements that may be made to them. There are different depths that one can be taken to. A relatively light trance, in which the individual is aware of what is happening to them, is suitable for behavioural work, such as treating anxiety and phobias. Deep trance is better suited for analytical work in order to help the individual solve deeper-held beliefs and to uncover deeply repressed memories.

It is important that in deeper work the individual is taken to a safe place in their mind where repressed memories and past experiences can be viewed in an objective manner, without producing any lingering distress. The skill and the qualification of the hypnotherapist are of paramount importance.

Many therapists who use hypnotherapy may incorporate other techniques and approaches like CBT and NLP into their treatment.

KEY POINTS

There are many types of talking therapies:

- Some are approved by NICE and are available free on the NHS in the UK
- Some analytical therapies may awaken deep memories and emotions and may make the individual feel worse for a while
- Qualifications vary widely – if seeking care privately, ask to check the qualifications and training of a therapist.

Chapter 9

Feeling desperate

The mind is its own place, and in itself, can make heaven of Hell, and a hell of Heaven.

John Milton (1608–1674), *Paradise Lost*

Sometimes emotions overwhelm us. When that happens it can be difficult to function. When people feel depressed, lacking in self-worth or feeling that there is no point in life, they may feel the need to self-harm.

Forms of self-harm

Self-harming can surface in many ways – not just the commonly thought-of methods such as taking an overdose of tablets or cutting yourself. Some sufferers will burn themselves, punch themselves or bang their heads against a wall. Some people will even swallow objects to cause pain and internal injury

The sufferer may feel that they are a cauldron of seething emotion and that they just need to take action, possibly taking tablets to end their life, or venting anger by hurting themselves. Some people do it a lot and keep it concealed from others, often appearing perfectly normal, cool and calm, while quietly hurting themselves. Others may do it in an outburst and draw attention to the fact. They may even have been working up to it, planning it some time in advance.

Most people who self-harm admit that they do it when they feel desperate, as a sort of coping mechanism. It is not, however, an effective coping mechanism, nor is it a helpful one.

Why do people self-harm?

This is a complex area and individual sufferers cannot be neatly pigeonholed. Some people repeatedly self-harm by cutting or scratching themselves because it is a way of venting anger, but in an internalised manner rather than having tantrums or harming someone else.

Some people do it to punish themselves and gain some ease from their emotion by causing themselves pain.

Others self-harm with the intention of killing themselves. All overdoses are serious as are all thoughts of ending your life by dramatic means, like jumping off a building, hanging yourself or throwing yourself under a train.

KEY POINTS

- Overdosing is the most common type of self-harm, accounting for 80 per cent of cases.
- Cutting is the second most common type, accounting for 15 per cent of cases.
- 1 in 3 people who self-harm will do it again the following year.
- 3 in 100 people who self-harm will eventually kill themselves.

Recognise that you need help

If you self-harm or contemplate self-harming then you should recognise it as a warning that you need help. Do not be afraid or feel ashamed about telling someone. If you feel so desperate that you need to hurt yourself in any of the ways that I have just mentioned, then talk to a good friend, a relative or, ideally, your doctor.

Sometimes talking with a friend or relative does not appeal because they are too close to you or you feel that they will not understand. Talking to a stranger who is skilled in listening may be appropriate, in which case there are several self-help agencies and support groups that offer telephone and Internet help. See Directory for more information.

Samaritans

This is a voluntary group which offers support 24 hours a day, seven days a week. It is non-religious and non-judgemental. You can call them at any time and speak to a volunteer. You can even email or arrange a face-to-face meeting.

The important thing to know is that you do not have to be suicidal to speak to them.

NHS Direct and NHS 111

NHS Direct was the original helpline offered by the National Health Service, but this is gradually being replaced with the new NHS 111 system. You can telephone at any time 24 hours a day, seven days a week with a concern and speak to an operator who will take details and will then hand you on to someone who can help. You may be advised of another service to contact in your locality.

The Silent Cry

This is a charity that was set up in 2008 to help people deal with self-harm and depression. Their website has videos and downloadable information.

Accident and Emergency Units

Your local Accident and Emergency Unit will always be a place that you can contact and attend if you feel desperate and if you have actually self-harmed. Indeed, if you have contacted your doctor, then you may be referred to the unit in the first instance.

What you can do yourself

In Part Three of the book I want to introduce you to a model that I call the Life Cycle, which can be adapted to deal with all sorts of problems, including when you feel desperate and want to self-harm. You will see how the things that I am going to talk about now can be incorporated into it.

Talk

This does not necessarily mean talk about how you are feeling, but just talk to someone. This can be a friend or relative who would be empathetic to your feelings, but if you think they are not, then just engage in talking. It will help to distract from the way that you are feeling. That process of distraction can sometimes be all that is needed to lessen the immediate feeling.

Be in the right place

Sometimes when you feel desperate the place that you are in or the people that you are with is actually part of the problem, as they may be triggering the desperate feelings. If so, try to go somewhere that feels better. That may involve going into a room with someone that you are more comfortable with, or perhaps visiting a friend.

Going off on your own or locking yourself in the bathroom may be entirely the wrong places, since they may be exactly where you would intend to self-harm yourself.

Distraction

Choose to do something different that will distract your thoughts. Put on a movie, listen to some uplifting music, go for a walk with the dog, or bake some bread. Aim to become calmer and focus on the pleasantness of being relaxed.

Substitution

Try substituting self-harm with something else that is not going to hurt you. For example, if you cut or scratch yourself then try substituting a pen for a blade. Draw on yourself. Using a red felt tip pen may help, as the mind may associate the red ink with the blood that would come from a cut. Another possibility is to apply a henna tattoo to the area that you would normally cut. Similarly, if you feel that you have to experience pain, then get some ice cubes and hold them tightly. The cold will soon cause pain, without causing long-term damage.

Do something nice

Do something nice for someone; it will help to take your mind away from the feelings that are driving you towards self-harm.

Reflect

After the feelings have subsided and you feel more yourself again and no longer feel that you want to self-harm, think about what it was that helped you get out of the mood and lose the sense of desperation. Was it a particular thing that you did, or a place that you went to or a person who you talked to? Focus and reflect on how you can incorporate any of those things into your life in future to prevent reoccurrences.

Chapter 10

Depression in children and young people

Children need models rather than critics.

Joseph Joubert (1754–1824), essayist

As recently as the 1980s it was assumed that children could not get depressed, because they lacked sufficient emotional maturity to feel low in mood. Equally, it was accepted that once they became teenagers they started to become confused by the outpouring of hormones and became moody.

Over the years, this perception has changed and an increasing number of children and adolescents are being treated for depression. Indeed, in the UK in 2003 over 50,000 children were prescribed antidepressants and over 170,000 prescriptions were given to people under the age of 18. Currently, it is estimated that up to 5 per cent of children and up to 20 per cent of adolescents are depressed.

Changing society

It may be that the increase in the numbers of children and young adults diagnosed with depression reflects the way that society has changed. It has in fact been a dramatic change over the last 60 years.

In the 1950s, children were generally brought up in a more disciplined and authoritarian culture, with the view that they would eventually go to work in order to help the country prosper. In the 1960s there came a change in society with more emphasis on permissiveness and freedom, and since then there has been an increasing trend towards pleasure-seeking consumerism. With a changing economy has come greater mobility, a breakdown of the extended family, increasing numbers of families where both parents work so less time is spent together and, of course, family break-ups have become more common.

There is an interesting effect from all this change. Increased consumerism has meant that there has been a strong trickle-down effect in which children have been allowed greater access to the adult world. They have computers, Internet access and mobile phones. Thus, the boundaries between childhood and adulthood have become blurred and children have become viewed as small adults. Because of this, it may be that moodiness and various behaviours that were once considered normal in teenagers are now considered abnormal and thereby deemed worthy of treatment.

This is not to say that children and young people do not become depressed. They quite clearly do, but as society changes so do the pressures that it puts upon people at the younger end of that society. Indeed, it may be that depression has become a catch-all diagnosis for unhappiness, sadness and moodiness. Since children tend to be regarded as little adults, one can see how the adult diagnosis has been extended to include children. This in part may explain why prescribing antidepressants for young people has increased.

Recognising depression in young people

Of course, you can turn things around and say that perhaps the numbers of children and young people who are depressed have always been the same, but in the past their depression was just not recognised. The important thing now, however, has to be the recognition of depression and giving whatever supports are needed, since there is good evidence that the earlier one feels depressed, the more likely it is to become chronic.

The symptoms of depression in children are not necessarily the same as with adults, partly because they may not have developed the language ability to communicate how they feel.

The signs of depression include:

- Generally unhappy demeanour
- Difficulty concentrating
- Very often weepy
- Recurrent physical symptoms, e.g. abdominal pain, headaches, fatigue
- Irritable or moody much of the time
- Tendency to be isolated and friendless
- Tendency to perform below their potential at school
- May be badly behaved
- May seem to be bullied
- May become a bully
- Loss of appetite and weight loss
- Loss of interest in things that previously interested them
- Low self-esteem
- Thoughts of self-harm.

Most parents do not like to think that their children could be depressed. Many of the reasons for adults not reporting their own depression may be at work here, for example the stigma, the fear that it could be a sign of mental weakness, worry about how others may think they are bringing their child up, or denial that there is a problem.

If you suspect that your child is depressed then seek advice from your GP.

Increased risk of depression in children and young people

Some children are more at risk than others. This can be risk from inherited factors or as a reaction to events in their life.

The following may be risk factors:

- If there is a family history of depression
- If there is a family history of suicide
- If there has been a bereavement
- If there has been a traumatic family background
- If there has been sexual or physical abuse
- If there has been bullying
- If there is a history of self-harm, e.g. scratching or cutting
- If they have been subject to neglect
- If they have had long-term problems with health
- If they have abused alcohol or drugs – do not discount this as many children are exposed to such things at an early age.

Seeking help

Your doctor is a good starting point, as always. He or she will almost certainly want to chat to your child to make an initial assessment. Then, if depression is suspected, a referral to the Community Mental Health Team is highly likely, or a referral to a paediatrician, who may have special knowledge. The important thing is to get the ball rolling. A series of psychological and medical tests may be arranged in order to help with the diagnosis and establish a management plan.

It is also a good idea to gather information by getting other members of the family to talk to your child, as talking will always help. Don't try to be therapists, but be supportive relatives. Much of the help here is in collecting other opinions and impressions that can be handed on to your doctor or to a member of the CMHT.

It is also a reasonable idea to contact support groups who may supply you with useful information and advice. See Directory for further information.

YoungMinds

This is a charity committed to improving the emotional wellbeing and mental health of children and young people. They have a Parents' Helpline and online resources that may be very useful.

Childline

This is a national helpline for young people. They can help with all sorts of problems such as self-harm and the reporting of sexual abuse.

Rethink Mental Illness

This is a national voluntary sector provider of mental health services, which offers information, advocacy and advice and has support groups throughout the country.

Treatment available

As with adult depression, three levels of depression are recognised.

Mild depression – when there is prolonged unhappiness, but the child is still able to lead a normal life.

Moderate depression – when the unhappiness is constant and deeper and it starts to impact on their life. Schoolwork may be affected and relationships may be strained. Your GP should certainly be consulted if this level of unhappiness is reached.

Severe depression – when the unhappiness is so bad that the child clearly is not coping or if they express the view that they are not coping. This has to be taken incredibly seriously, because the child may have suicidal thoughts but not be verbalising them to anyone.

For each level of depression, the following treatments may be put in place:

Talking therapies

Mainly, the treatment emphasis is with talking therapies. These may be individual therapies like counselling, or more in depth like Cognitive Behavioural Therapy (CBT – to help change negative ways of thinking), Interpersonal Therapy (IPT – to explore relationships) or family therapy (in which the whole family is involved in the care).

Antidepressants

Some children with severe depression may be prescribed antidepressants. This is likely to be one of the Selective Serotonin Reuptake Inhibitor, SSRI group of drugs. These will generally be on the advice of a consultant psychiatrist. These have been shown to be the safest and most effective at this age.

Monitoring

The vast majority of children and young people will be managed in the community without having to be admitted to hospital. It is only if self-harm or suicidal thoughts are present that hospital admission would be likely.

Follow-ups would generally take place on a weekly basis for four weeks, then at regular intervals until recovery has taken place.

KEY POINTS

- 2 per cent of children under 12 years are depressed
- 5 per cent of teenagers are depressed
- More than half of adults who become depressed say that they had depressed moods before they were 20 years old
- Symptoms lasting more than three weeks may be significant and advice should be sought from your GP
- If a child ever talks about suicide consider it a danger signal and seek help and advice promptly
- Most cases of childhood depression will have settled after about eight months
- There is an increasing rate of suicide in younger adult males

Chapter 11

Depression in older age

Anyone who stops learning is old, whether at twenty or eighty. Anyone who keeps learning stays young. The greatest thing in life is to keep your mind young.

Henry Ford (1863–1947), American industrialist and businessman

> ## Depression is not a normal part of getting old

Many people experience depression in old age as they become less mobile and more prone to illness. It is a time in life when one has to deal with lots of changes. Retirement can bring with it a feeling of loss, as you no longer have the discipline of a work routine, or the pressure to earn a living and support a family. It is easy to feel that life has less of a purpose after retirement, which can lead to lower self-esteem. Not only that, but isolation and loneliness may have to be dealt with, as well as the possibility of bereavement as loved ones and friends may pass away.

While you may feel that there are more reasons to feel down as you enter the Third Age of life, it doesn't mean that being melancholic is a natural part of growing old. There are many things that can be done to tackle depression in older age, but first you need to be able to identify it.

How common is it?

Depression in the elderly is surprisingly common and its incidence rises with age.

- 15 per cent of over-65s suffer from depression.

- 30 per cent of over-75s suffer from depression.

- Only about 30 per cent of elderly depression sufferers are known to their doctors; it is likely that this figure is so low because many of the people expect to have to put up with this as they get older.

Depression is not something that one should just accept, since it is not a function of ageing. And indeed, depression puts people at risk of suicide.

KEY POINTS

- Depression is not a normal part of ageing.
- Depression puts people at risk of suicide.
- Males over the age of 75 have the highest suicide rates in most industrialised countries (although there is an increasing suicide rate among younger males in their 20s).
- In the elderly, depression is the most important predictor of suicide.
- Widowed elderly men have three times the risk as elderly men still married.

Difficulty of diagnosis

The first difficulty is that sufferers often do not complain about their depression. If you are immobilised or incapacitated by a physical condition then the signs that something is not right are obvious, but feeling depressed may not seem to have the same impact, and relatives and friends may not be aware of it. People may put your irritability simply down to old age when in fact you may be feeling miserable.

As with children and young people, the classic signs of depression are not always obvious in the elderly and symptoms may just be attributed to age and therefore accepted by the person and their family. There will probably be low mood and there may be accompanying difficulty with thinking and concentrating. There may also be some disturbance of appetite and a tendency to wake early in the mornings. Sadness and tearfulness are obvious signs, but there may be more subtle signs, such as becoming more anxious, or becoming neglectful of oneself.

The following are indications of depression in the elderly:

- Sadness

- Fatigue

- Sleep difficulties

- Poor self-esteem

- Difficulty concentrating

- Memory problems

- Preoccupation with death and dying

- Suicidal thoughts

- Increased use of alcohol

- Loss of interest in hobbies

- Self-neglect

- Loss of appetite and weight loss

- Self-isolation.

It is common for a feeling of sadness or melancholy to be present, but it is not always apparent. Indeed, sometimes the sufferer is not aware that they are depressed because they do not feel sad. Physical symptoms may be more dominant, or they may just feel that they can't be bothered with things. They may have a lack of motivation and energy, and simply attribute them to age. Yet they may be depressed.

KEY POINT

Depression in the elderly may not always manifest itself as sadness or feeling down.

Risk factors

Stiff upper lip

Some people reach an age when they think that people don't want to hear about their feelings and their psychological symptoms, even when they themselves know that they are feeling depressed. The 'stiff upper lip' may be concealing depression that could be treated to make them feel better.

Physical illness

Severe ongoing physical illness has been found to be a major risk factor for depression in old age. One research study showed that 60 per cent of elderly depressed patients were suffering from serious physical illness, which interfered with their daily life. The most significant physical illnesses seem to be strokes and heart attacks. Partly, this seems to be because they limit mobility and cause dependence upon others. Also, these conditions often give people the feeling that they are living on the brink of a volcano – they are waiting for the next one to happen. As a result, they become depressed. A history of cancer is also commonly associated with depression, since there may be anxiety that it will come back and that it could kill them.

Other chronic conditions may not be life-threatening, but are associated with depression. This can be a direct effect of the condition, or it can be a psychological reaction to it. The following are associated with depression, and treatment of the condition may improve the depression: Parkinson's disease, chronic arthritis, diabetes, multiple sclerosis, thyroid disorders, vitamin B12 deficiency and anaemia and Alzheimer's disease.

Social change and loss

These are potentially very important. After all, the loss of loved ones and friends becomes more common, and the sense of loneliness and isolation becomes more acute. The thought: 'I'm the only one left' may make the individual aware of their own mortality. Fear of that can be enough to develop depression.

Housing problems, money worries and loss of resources can all be potent causes of depression, particularly if they have to be coped with alone.

Pets may be a lifeline to the elderly and the loss of a cat or a dog can cause just as significant a grief reaction as that of a person.

Fear can also trigger depression. We talked about anticipatory fear in the section on logotherapy. Well, this is again quite relevant, because the individual may fear death or fear the consequences of what their death may mean to the family. Fear of illness or financial difficulties can all create an empty feeling, which can result in depression.

Alcohol

This may be an issue that has to be handled delicately, if the person seems to be developing a habit or leaning too much on alcohol. It has to be understood that alcohol is a drug and a depressant drug at that. People often imagine that it lifts the mood. In fact, it does not. What happens is that it depresses brain cell functioning. The first brain cells that are depressed by it are the inhibitory neurones, which are the last ones to be developed as we grow up and develop social skills. Their function is to stop us doing unsocial things. So, when you have a little alcohol these neurones are depressed and the mood seems to improve and the person seems to relax and 'let their hair down'. Imbibing a bit more will result in yet more brain cells being depressed and the individual may do increasingly unsocial things. Even more alcohol and the motor brain cells, which control body movements, are depressed. One slurs, becomes unsteady and the state of drunkenness is reached.

Long-term alcohol intake still depresses brain cells, but may lead to depression. Also, if someone is taking prescription drugs, there could well be an interaction between the alcohol and the drugs that may induce iatrogenic depression.

This is not to say that one should avoid alcohol, but responsible and moderate drinking is the answer.

Grief and depression

Since bereavements become more common the older one gets, we need to consider this in a little more detail here. Sometimes an older person may seem to simply take a long time to get over a loss. In that case, they may not be suffering from grief, but may have fallen into a depression.

There are several recognised stages of grief. Generally, a normal grief process lasts for about three months. There will still be emotional pain, but things will become easier after that.

The following are the normal grief stages:

Initial shock

The person cannot accept that the person has gone; they may even exhibit the mental mechanism of 'denial' whereby they refuse to believe that the person has died. This shock is often accompanied by emotional blunting, so that the person does not weep as much as they would expect, or they just cannot cry.

Yearning

This comes after a few days. The person yearns and wants the deceased person to come back. They find themselves filled with memories and images. They want to be close to their things and personal effects. In this time, which can last for a week or two, there is often anger that the person has been taken away, that certain people did not do enough, and so on. The anger is not usually justified. Then there is guilt; perhaps if only they had done certain things the individual would still be with them, or they feel guilt about things that had or had not been said before the person died.

Despair

This can last a few more weeks. This is the sadness that comes when it is realised that person has gone. It is common for people to hibernate, to become apathetic and to feel that life is pointless.

Recovery

The main hurting starts to go. It is a matter of coming to terms with the loss so that you can start to rebuild your life.

After three months or so, the individual can expect to see some return of joy. Watching a TV show may induce a laugh, or a hug from a friend or relative may make them feel better. If not, then the grief may have developed into depression.

If any of the listed symptoms above appear at this time then depression is likely. In particular, if the person starts having thoughts about suicide, or if they feel racked with guilt, then they may need help.

Things that may help one to grieve

It is helpful to try to maintain some sense of normality in your life during grief or loss.

People usually offer help initially, but if their help is declined they may not offer it again. Try not to be reticent, but accept help when it is offered and, indeed, do not be afraid to ask family and friends.

Try to get into a routine every day. If you languish into a chaotic pattern then it is easy to lose purpose, and when one loses a sense of purpose depression can result.

Try not to resort to alcohol, for it does not actually help. It is easy to become dependent on it and to develop a habit that ultimately you do not need and which can contribute to depression, as mentioned earlier.

Accept that the emotions you are feeling are normal, and that if you feel like weeping, allow yourself to do so.

Look after yourself and make sure that you get some exercise and that you have regular nutritious meals, both of which will help.

Dementia and depression

Many of the symptoms of depression can be attributed to the person undergoing some degree of cognitive impairment. Memory problems, difficulty in concentrating and slowness of thinking may be attributed to 'senior moments'. Relatives may even assume that it is the beginning of Alzheimer's disease. The presence of any of these signs should be taken seriously for two reasons. Firstly, it could be depression that would be amenable to treatment. Secondly, if it is a cognitive problem then the sooner it is looked at and investigated the better. Treatment for that may help.

In addition, even if it is a cognitive problem, then depression could still be present and the treatment of the depression could improve the cognitive function.

The following may help to differentiate the two:

- The memory difficulty that is characteristic of dementia is loss of short-term memory.

- Mental decline in thought processes is slow and gradual in dementia, but may seem to have occurred rapidly in depression.

- In dementia there will usually be disorientation for time, date and where the person is. This is not a feature of depression.

Diogenes syndrome

This is a relatively rare yet important condition. It is named after Diogenes (412–323 BC), an ancient Greek philosopher who founded the Cynics discipline of philosophy. He had been a pupil of Antisthenes, who in turn had been a follower of Socrates. Upon Socrates' death Antisthenes rejected philosophy, thinking that it was useless quibbling and that man's sole concern should be to be good.

Diogenes adopted this life of austerity and lived in a barrel, like a dog. The word 'cynic' did not have its current meaning, but meant canine, or dog-like.

The person with Diogenes syndrome neglects themself and starts to hoard all manner of useless things. This can be newspapers, bags of rubbish, old bottles, etc. They will tend to withdraw from society and are at risk of malnutrition, anaemia and other problems that can result from self-neglect. There are treatments for it, and it does not mean that someone is suffering from a dementia process.

Iatrogenic depression

As mentioned in Chapter 2, 'iatrogenic' means 'caused by treatment'.

The elderly tend to be more sensitive to drugs than younger people, partly because their organs (especially the liver and kidneys) are gradually becoming less efficient. The list of drugs that can cause iatrogenic depression is substantial, and since the elderly are more likely to be on such drugs, this always needs to be taken into consideration. This is particularly important if someone starts to feel depressed soon after starting a new drug. Simply changing the drug may make a huge difference.

Psychosis in the elderly

Many elderly people experience psychotic symptoms of hallucinations and delusions at some point. These do not necessarily mean that they have a psychotic illness, however. For example, the Charles Bonnet syndrome is characterised by visual hallucinations accompanying deterioration of vision in the elderly. It usually resolves itself after a while. It is not a psychotic illness.

Delirium

This is also referred to as an acute confusional state. It is characterised by confused thinking, disorientation, which may be for time and place – in that they are unsure if it is day or night, or where they are. This is often confused with dementia, so it is important to investigate it; it may have a cause, such as a urinary infection, a deficiency state or a problem with hormones, that may be treatable with good results.

Having said that, the two can co-exist, but even if dementia is present, treating a toxic state should help.

Paraphrenia or psychosis in the elderly

This is a psychotic state in which the person may be depressed, but the overriding feature is the presence of paranoid delusions. Memory and thought processes may be otherwise intact.

Similar to delirium, it may co-exist with dementia. Good diagnosis and treatment may make a big difference to both the depression and the delusions.

Treatment of depression in the elderly

Drug treatment is just as effective for the elderly as it is for younger groups. As mentioned earlier, other medical conditions may be contributing to the depression, either as part of the nature of the condition, or as a psychological result.

The choice of antidepressant drug is a matter for your doctor to decide. It should be mentioned that the dosage might not need to be as high as with younger people, because the individual may be more sensitive to drugs.

Also, the SSRI group of drugs, which we looked at in Chapter 7, have been shown to cause rapid bone loss and therefore there is a higher risk of fractures. These drugs should be carefully monitored.

If psychotic depression or paraphrenia is present, then this may well necessitate hospital treatment and the use of antipsychotic medication.

Other strategies may be needed to help depression, including exercise. This is beneficial to everyone, and no one is ever too old to start exercising. Even if someone has restricted mobility, there are always safe exercises that can be done in a chair or on a bed. Your doctor can advise on this or arrange for help from a physiotherapist or occupational therapist.

Social supports are important and every effort should be made to avoid isolation. Joining clubs or going to care centres where one can be with other people can make a huge difference.

The sufferer should be encouraged to get good sleep, since insufficient sleep can lead to depression. It is best to avoid sleeping tablets or alcohol, however.

Similarly, diet should be looked at. It is important to have an adequate diet with plenty of fruit and vegetables and adequate protein. It is important to avoid too much sugar, fried foods and junk food, as they can all lead to depression. The exact reasons why are still not clear, but sugary food can affect the blood sugar levels, which go up and down like a yo-yo and can have an effect on the blood vessels of the brain. In addition, they tend to increase the likelihood of inflammation, so many physical conditions can be worsened.

It may also be that one or other of the talking therapies will be suggested. This is especially likely if the person has had a trauma, such as a bereavement, and they need some help in working through it.

Help from family and neighbours

It is not always easy to consider the needs of elderly people living alone when people have busy lives themselves. The thought that someone is at home, with no work to do and plenty of time to potter about and watch TV, may make relatives and neighbours think that they are safe and happy. Yet as we have discussed, that is not necessarily the case. They may be depressed, and if they are depressed they may be at risk of suicide.

Showing concern and offering help can make a big difference to someone who is depressed. Offering to take them out, to help with their social needs and helping them to maintain social contacts can literally be life-saving.

Making sure that elderly friends or relatives have regular meals, that they are taking their medication regularly and are not neglecting themselves, can all help prevent depression.

And, most importantly, communicating and asking how they are feeling is essential. If they express symptoms of depression, especially if they talk about feeling useless or that life has no meaning, then they may be thinking about suicide. It is a real risk as mentioned earlier, so get some medical help as soon as possible.

Chapter 12

Postnatal depression

To give birth is a fearsome thing; there is no hating the child one has borne even when injured by it.

Sophocles (497–406 BC), Greek playwright

Giving birth to a child is a major event in a woman's life. It brings great responsibility as well as great joy. Yet it is common for women to experience low mood at some stage after the birth. This can range from baby blues, which is extremely common, short-lived and quite normal, to postnatal depression (PND) which can be very distressing and which needs treatment, to postpartum psychosis, which is rare and needs specialist psychiatric treatment.

Baby blues

This is a mild mood disturbance that is experienced by half to two-thirds of all mothers. It is most common in first-time mothers and in women who have a history of moderate-to-severe premenstrual syndrome. It seems to be related to the rapid change in hormones that occur as the body readjusts after birth.

It usually starts on the third or fourth day after the birth. The mother may experience mood swings, sadness, anxiety and tearfulness. It may last for up to a week, but most women find that it disappears by day ten. It requires no treatment other than reassurance.

Postnatal depression

This is a depressive illness that affects between 10 and 15 per cent of mothers. There is a feeling of sadness, vulnerability and any of the other symptoms that we have considered.

Postnatal depression can follow on from baby blues or it can develop later, usually within the first month after birth, although it can even develop several months after the birth. It is considered to be present if the symptoms have lasted for more than two weeks. About one-third of women with postnatal depression actually start to become depressed during their pregnancy and continue after they give birth.

Like depression at other stages of life, it can vary in severity from mild to moderate and severe. One can cope and manage with mild postnatal depression, but when it is moderate to severe it can be difficult to cope with both yourself and the baby.

Common symptoms are:

Depressed mood – The woman feels unhappy and miserable for a lot of the time.

Weepy – There may be tearfulness for a lot of the time, with sudden bursts of tears for no obvious reason.

No pleasure – Feeling unable to derive any joy from anything, including possibly the new baby.

Irritability – This may be with one's partner, but may also be with other children and the new baby.

Sleep problems – This can be extremely debilitating, since it may be hard to get off to sleep.

Fatigue and lack of energy – This can be so bad that simple things prove difficult. It may be related to sleep problems, but can occur in the absence of them.

Anxiety – This is extremely common. Most mothers are anxious about their baby's health. That is normal. In postnatal depression these anxieties may dominate one's life:

- Fear that the baby is ill
- Worry about the baby being small or not putting on weight
- Worry that the baby will not settle
- Worry that everyone will think she is a bad mother
- Worry that the baby might have a cot death
- Worry that she could harm the baby
- Worry about one's own health
- Despair that the depression will never end
- Worry that the baby could be taken away from them.

This anxiety can manifest as physical symptoms like butterflies in the tummy, palpitations, sweating, increased looseness of the bowels, breathlessness and even faintness.

The anxiety about harming the baby is common in postnatal depression, but actually harming is quite rare. Most people who have these thoughts do not follow them through. If a woman does have them at all then she should talk about it with the health visitor and her GP.

Following on from this is the anxiety that the baby could be taken away from her. This may make some women fearful of telling anyone how they feel, in case they are considered a danger to their child. In fact, the health visitor and the GP are on her side. They will do all that can be done to help and if further help is needed from the CMHT, then it will be arranged.

Poor self-esteem – Feeling unworthy and hopeless is common. So too is feeling ugly and unattractive. There may be a tendency to isolate oneself and avoid going out.

Appetite changes – Some women lose their appetite and have trouble eating. Others may binge and put weight on.

Libido loss – It is common in postnatal depression to lose any sexual desire. Some women feel that they do not want to be touched or hugged.

Guilt – This is quite common. The mother may feel bad about not loving her baby, or about not looking after the baby or her other children. There may be guilt about not wanting her partner near her or it can spill over into other areas in life. The thing is that the guilt is almost never justified. It is a useless emotion that simply makes you feel worse.

Suicidal thoughts – This is a danger signal and you should seek help immediately. If someone at risk verbalises this to you, you should immediately seek help from their health visitor or GP.

Risk factors for PND

It is not usually possible to say why postnatal depression occurs. It may be a combination of factors coupled with the changes in hormone levels. A review of the literature in 2010 was published in the *American Journal of Obstetrics and Gynaecology*.[9] It showed that the following factors put a woman at risk of developing postnatal depression:

- Anxiety tendency

- Stress in life during the pregnancy

- Past depression

- Lack of social support

- Domestic violence and abuse

- Unplanned pregnancy

- Relationship problems.

Dealing with PND

The first thing is to acknowledge that there is a problem. You should not be worried about telling your health visitor or your GP that you are feeling depressed. No one will think any the less of you for doing so and there is almost no question about your baby being taken away from you.

Recent research by the universities of Leicester, Nottingham and Sheffield, published in 2010, has shown that health visitors trained in giving psychological support reduce the risk of developing postnatal depression by 30 per cent. Therefore, maintaining a close relationship with your health visitor is very beneficial.

You should also try to help yourself by giving yourself more time. Don't think that you have to be able to do all the things that you did before you fell pregnant. Your baby needs more time, so let some commitments go.

Try to eat and sleep regularly and accept help wherever and whenever it is offered.

Be as sociable as you can. Talking with and being with other new mothers helps, because it shows that you are not on your own. You will probably find other women who have had similar experiences and their advice may help a great deal.

It is also possible to use computerised Cognitive Behavioural Therapy (see p. 101).

Talking therapies

Talking therapies may be needed if the PND is more severe. Your doctor will arrange this, perhaps with a counsellor, either at the medical practice or at another centre. Your health visitor may even be able to offer this, especially if she has had additional psychological training as mentioned above.

Cognitive Behavioural Therapy can be arranged with the CMHT. This will focus on looking at and helping you change the way you think and behave, and seeing things differently.

Other talking therapies like interpersonal psychotherapy may be appropriate, perhaps focusing on relationships. Your doctor will advise on this.

Antidepressants

These may be needed and your doctor will prescribe the right one for you. If you are breast-feeding then certain ones are not used, because they can find their way into the breast milk. It may even be that breast-feeding difficulties have been a factor in the postnatal depression and a decision to stop breast-feeding may remove the pressure that the mother puts upon herself. In that case, other antidepressants may be considered.

The older tricyclic antidepressants are used less frequently than the SSRI drugs. Of the SSRIs, sertraline and paroxetine are the favoured choice in breast-feeding mothers.

Postpartum psychosis

This is a rarer but serious condition, which affects one mother in every thousand after birth. It is quite different from postnatal depression and it necessitates help as soon as possible. It has several other names including puerperal psychosis, postnatal psychosis and postpartum onset bipolar disorder.

In the UK, 1,300 women experience postpartum psychosis every year.

The symptoms are variable. They may be depression symptoms, which can be extremely severe, or they can be feelings of intense elation and mania. There may be agitation and restlessness. There may also be detachment from reality manifesting as delusions and hallucinations.

A delusion is a false idea that becomes fixed in the person's mind and which they cannot be reasoned out of. For example, that they are someone else, or that the baby is not theirs.

Hallucinations occur when the person sees things (visual hallucination) or hears voices (auditory hallucination) that are not real.

Other symptoms include:

- Feeling elated

- Pressure of thought – the thoughts race

- Extreme talkativeness

- Depression

- Thoughts seem slow or seem to get blocked

- Confusion

- Anxiety irritability

- Hostility

- Suspiciousness

- Withdrawing from everyone

- Sleep problems, including losing the desire to sleep

- Paranoia – when it seems that everyone is talking about the person

- Erratic and odd behaviour.

These symptoms can develop within hours of having the baby, or any time up to a couple of weeks afterwards.

All of these are potentially serious symptoms and help is needed as soon as possible. A psychiatrist will be asked to see the mother and he or she will arrange and monitor treatment.

The cause is not known

Whereas in postnatal depression there may be an obvious trigger, this is not usually the case in postpartum psychosis. It seems to simply come out of the blue. It is not caused by faulty or difficult relationships and it is not because of anything that the mother may have done. It is a cloudy area and more research needs to be done on it.

Risk factors for postpartum psychosis

Postpartum psychosis is most common in first pregnancies. The risk is increased if there has been:

- A previous episode of severe depression

- A family history of serious mental illness, including both depression and schizophrenia

- A previous episode of a psychotic illness or bipolar depression

- Complications during delivery of the baby

- A postpartum psychosis in a previous pregnancy – there is a high risk of having another episode in another pregnancy. This can be anything between a 1 in 4 and a 1 in 2 chance.

For women at high risk

If a woman is at high risk and is trying to conceive, it is important that she should alert her doctor and her psychiatrist. This is important in terms of medication and the risk that it could have to a developing baby.

The CMHT, the midwife and the obstetric team should all be made aware of the risk so that she can be given the help that she needs during pregnancy, through the delivery and through the postnatal period.

It is desirable to have a pre-birth meeting at about 32 weeks of pregnancy. This should include everyone involved in the care of the patient and, of course, includes the mother-to-be and her family. A care plan should be prepared, with a list of how to access help and from whom.

In hospital, the midwifery and obstetric staff will give whatever care is needed and a psychiatrist will see the mother during that time and any medication will be monitored.

On discharge, part of the management plan should include emergency numbers for the CMHT or the crisis team.

Of course, being at high risk of having an episode does not mean that one will occur, and if appropriate care and attention have been taken it is to be hoped that it can be avoided.

Treatment of postpartum psychosis

If postpartum psychosis does occur then it is likely that hospital treatment will be needed and, ideally, this should take place in a Mother and Baby Unit. These units are specially designed for mothers with such a problem and are where the mother and baby can be admitted and cared for, and the mother treated while they are there. This is the most desirable situation.

If such a unit is not available locally then the mother will need to be admitted to a ward in a psychiatric hospital. This will mean that the baby will have to be cared for by the partner or the mother's family. Social Services may be able to help and find a temporary carer if that is not possible.

Medication

This will be different from postnatal depression, since antidepressants are probably not going to be sufficient on their own. It is likely that patients will need an antipsychotic drug and perhaps a mood stabiliser. Sometimes both might be needed.

This is essentially the same sort of treatment that is needed with other psychotic illnesses. The only difference is that if the mother is breast-feeding, then the selection of drugs needs to be made on the basis that they do not interfere with the breast-feeding or pass into the milk.

Social Services

Some women may be referred to Children and Families Social Services. This can be alarming, but it is not in order to remove children into care but to ensure that the needs of the child are being taken care of. That is, it may be necessary to see that further care is made available if the mother and the family are struggling.

This would be discussed with the mother in the first instance.

Prognosis

'Prognosis' means 'outlook'. Generally, with postpartum psychosis it is a good outlook with the vast majority of mothers recovering fully.

The worse symptoms take from two weeks to three months to settle, and it can take anything from six months to a year to recover fully from postpartum psychosis. Having said that, it is not unusual to experience further episodes of depression. In part, this can relate to the fact that postpartum psychosis occurs when a mother should be enjoying the early stages of being with and bonding with her newborn baby. Bonding does usually take place, but it can just be delayed.

As mentioned above, subsequent pregnancies carry a higher risk of having an episode and a good management plan and close liaison between GP, midwife, obstetric staff and psychiatrist is needed.

Helpful organisations

There are several useful groups and organisations that invite enquiries and advice, which people with postnatal depression and postpartum psychosis may find of value. See Directory for further information.

Action Postpartum Psychosis Network

This is a network of women across the UK who have experienced postpartum psychosis, run in collaboration with academics experts from Birmingham and Cardiff Universities. Among other things, they can offer leaflets and information for women and their families, an online PPtalk forum where women and families can talk with women who have suffered with it and a peer support network where contacts can be suggested.

Association for Postnatal Illness (APNI)

This Association provides a telephone helpline, information and leaflets for sufferers from postnatal illness and a network of volunteers who have suffered from postnatal illness.

Cry-sis

A helpline offering self-help advice and support to parents with excessively crying and demanding babies.

PANDAS

An online community supporting people with antenatal and postnatal depression. They can provide a call line for support, a letter service for those who prefer to express themselves in writing or an email service, and can put you in touch with a support group.

Chapter 13

Treatment-resistant depression

Fall seven times, stand up eight.

Japanese proverb

Some people do not respond well to antidepressant medication. If they do not respond to at least two antidepressants then they may have treatment-resistant depression or TRD. It is sometimes also referred to as treatment-refractory depression. The term was first used in 1974 and the treatment advised by psychiatrists at that time was to have a course of electro-convulsive therapy (ECT). Things have progressed considerably since then and there are different strategies that can be called upon.

It isn't getting any better

It can be a harrowing experience to find that the recommended treatment fails to bring about any improvement in how you are feeling. It can serve to reinforce the sense of helplessness and hopelessness that you may already be experiencing.

Most people with depression who take antidepressants or who engage in one or other of the talking therapies will improve. One in three people with depression, however, will not respond to the first course of antidepressants. They are likely to respond to subsequent ones. Yet up to 20 per cent of people who experience depression will go on to have chronic depression that will seem to defy treatments.

Treatment-resistant depression can range from mild to severe and several approaches may be needed. It is a diagnosis that usually means that a consultant psychiatrist will need to be involved, along with other members of the CMHT.

There is growing evidence that combining pharmacological or drug therapy with talking therapy may very well help. This is the advice of the National Institute for Health and Care Excellence.

Antidepressants

The thing is not to despair if an antidepressant is not doing the trick straight away. Remember that an antidepressant probably will not start to function until you have been on it for 10–14 days. It then sometimes needs some adjustment of the dose; and then if that doesn't work, another course of a different one is reasonable.

Augmentation

Some people need to have two different types of antidepressant prescribed at the same time. This may be done by your own GP. This is called augmentation of one drug with another to get a combined effect.

The tricyclic-like drug mianserin is recommended by NICE as a suitable antidepressant to augment the SSRI antidepressants. Blood tests need to be done, however, since there is a risk that the combination could result in agranulocytosis, a condition in which the white blood cell levels drop dramatically, which can make the patient susceptible to infection. It is a serious condition and a serious risk.

Patients should also be made aware of the risks of serotonin syndrome (see Chapter 7) with the SSRI antidepressants. They should certainly not take herbal preparations like St John's wort or ginseng at the same time, because of this potential problem.

If someone has failed to respond to augmentation, then referral to a psychiatrist would be reasonable.

Combining with CBT

A recent trial called the CoBalT trial randomised 469 patients with treatment-resistant depression, defined by them as having symptoms despite having taken an antidepressant for six weeks. They were randomised into two groups, one of which would only receive an antidepressant, while the other group would receive an antidepressant together with an additional course of CBT.[10] They found that the patients who received the CBT were three times more likely to experience a 50 per cent reduction in depressive symptoms than the patients who simply had antidepressants.

NICE now recommend that treatment-resistant patients should receive both an antidepressant and a course of CBT. They also recommend that if someone relapses while taking a course of antidepressants they should receive a course of CBT alongside the antidepressant.

Lithium augmentation

Lithium is a mood-stabiliser and NICE recommend that if a patient has not responded to several courses of antidepressants, and is still eager for help, then they should be prescribed a course of lithium augmentation. This means taking daily lithium in addition to a course of antidepressants. It will necessitate regular blood tests to check that the lithium level does not rise too high and that the kidney function is unimpaired.

The patient needs to be aware of the possible side effects (see Chapter 7). An ECG should be done before starting on lithium.

Venlafaxine

NICE also recommend that this drug should be considered in patients who have not responded to two adequate courses of antidepressants. The dose should be increased slowly under supervision, according to the recommended *British National Formulary* (BNF) limits. The patient should be warned about side effects, which can include palpitations, constipation, weight changes, insomnia, glaucoma, tinnitus and other problems (For a full list see the current *British National Formulary*; this is an annual joint publication by the British Medical Association and the Royal Pharmaceutical Society of Great Britain which has up-to-date information on medicines).

The patient should not stop taking the drug too quickly, because withdrawal effects can occur which can be unpleasant. Reduction should be done slowly under medical supervision.

Monoamine oxidase inhibitors (MAOIs)

These drugs are not used so much these days, yet they still have a second-line role in the treatment of several conditions, including treatment-resistant depression.

NICE recommend that the MAOI phenelzine could be used in patients who have failed to respond to other antidepressants and who are prepared to tolerate its side effects and the dietary restrictions that are associated with it. This essentially means avoiding tyramine-containing foods, such as cheese, pickles and broad beans, as well as processed foods.

Aspirin and the Cytokine Hypothesis

There is mounting evidence that depression could be related to inflammation.

A series of studies around the world strongly support the theory that cytokines can contribute to some cases of depression. This has been shown in studies carried out in Brighton, Glasgow, Bristol and King's College London, by members of PRIME, the Psychiatric Research into Inflammation, Immunity and Mood Effects, a consortium of UK researchers.

Two recent studies also showed that when people have been given medication for Hepatitis C and vaccination against typhoid, they became depressed. Here again, these are conditions associated with inflammation, and it backs up the Cytokine Hypothesis.

A specific trial by Dr Julien Mendlewicz from the Department of Psychiatry at Erasme Hospital in Belgium showed that when an SSRI antidepressant was augmented by aspirin in patients with treatment-resistant depression, the response rate to the antidepressant was increased substantially and the period of remission from depression was extended.[11]

More research needs to be done, but the PRIME collaboration suggests that the evidence is strong enough to justify prescribing aspirin or other anti-inflammatory drugs to augment antidepressants.

Other treatments

If drug treatment and CBT have not helped then the following treatments may be considered.

Electro-Convulsive Therapy (ECT)

When I began to work in psychiatry in the mid-1970s, prior to becoming a General Practitioner, ECT was used far more frequently than it is today. At that time, we had less effective drugs and ECT was seen as a useful treatment for what we would now consider major depression. In the psychiatric unit that I worked in we had a weekly ECT clinic where several patients would be treated. It has to be said that its use has always been controversial. Nowadays it is used only half as often as it was in 1985.

ECT is a treatment that involves delivering an electric current to the brain in order to produce a convulsion, or an epileptic fit. The rationale goes back to the days before there were any effective treatments for any mental illness, when it was noted that people with schizophrenia or depression who happened to also have epilepsy often reported that they felt better after having a fit.

ECT was developed in the 1930s and found wide usage. It was suggested that the fits somehow 'purged' the brain and jolted it back into a normal pattern. It was found that some patients reported significant memory loss afterwards and so various types of ECT were practised:

- Bilateral – the shock was delivered to both hemispheres of the brain.

- Unilateral, dominant – the shock was delivered to the dominant hemisphere of the brain, according to the handedness of the person.

- Unilateral non-dominant – the shock was delivered to the non-dominant hemisphere of the brain, according to the handedness of the person.

Bilateral ECT seemed to cause the most problems.

The fact is that we are uncertain how ECT works although it certainly does seem to be effective in a small group of patients. NICE suggest that its use should be restricted to major depression that is life-threatening, when other treatments have failed, in resistant mania and in catatonia (when the individual is totally immobilised and stuporose as a result of a psychiatric problem).

It is important to know that no one can be made to have ECT, even if they are admitted to hospital under a section of the Mental Health Act. It has to be a voluntarily accepted treatment.

Vagus nerve stimulation

This process involves implanting a device under the skin of the chest which is connected to the vagus nerve – the body's tenth cranial nerve – in the neck. Electrical signals from the device stimulate the vagus nerve and affect the mood centres in the brain. This is a treatment that has been used successfully for epilepsy and it has been called the 'pacemaker for the brain'.

This technique is still being investigated regarding its efficacy. In their information leaflet about this, *Vagus nerve stimulation for treatment-resistant depression*, published in 2009, NICE state that there is not much good evidence about how well this procedure works or how safe it is. Yet it has its advocates and some clinics may still advise having the procedure performed.

NICE mention an analysis of 18 studies including 1,251 patients who had it performed, in which 58 per cent had a satisfactory response lasting 12 months or more. In addition, another study of 74 patients with severe depression had the procedure and a 55 per cent success rate was recorded after one year.

Those figures may make it seem worth trying for someone who has been diagnosed with treatment-resistant depression.

> Leaflets and the full guidance for 'vagus nerve stimulation for treatment-resistant depression' aimed at healthcare professionals are available at ww.nice.org.uk/IPG330

Transcranial magnetic stimulation

This is a treatment that involves using electromagnetic fields to alter brain activity to help treatment-resistant depression. A large electromagnetic coil is held against the scalp near the forehead and an electric current is produced that flows through the brain. It is reported to be effective, but once again there is still not a lot of evidence.

At the moment this is not available on the NHS and one can only be offered it as part of a research study.

Again, NICE have produced a leaflet explaining the current position about it, aimed at healthcare professionals, which is available at www.nice.org.uk/IPG242.

Part Three

WHAT YOU CAN DO FOR YOURSELF

Dealing with depression is not about being the recipient of a treatment. There is much that the individual can do to help and to maintain their sense of wellbeing.

Chapter 14

The Life Cycle

Do not dwell in the past, do not dream of the future, concentrate the mind on the present moment.

Siddhārtha Gautama Buddha

We have covered a lot of ground in this book and it can be difficult for someone actually experiencing depression to know where to start in order to help themselves. In my own practice, I use a model that I call the Life Cycle to help patients to examine their life in order to devise strategies that they can use for self-help. I do not pretend that this is any kind of rocket science. It is simply a model that many people find useful to help them gain a bit of focus.

This term, 'life cycle', may take you back to your days of studying biology when you looked at the different life cycles of insects, fish, frogs and other creatures on the evolutionary ladder. I am not, however, using the term here in the same sense. I am using it as a model for a person's life. This has nothing to do with their development with age, but is to do with the different levels or spheres that make up one's life at any point in time. You will see that there is a cycle involved, certainly in the manner in which a condition

– virtually any chronic medical condition, whether that is a physical one or a psychological one like depression – can affect them.

To stay with the biology analogy a little longer, it can definitely be useful to study animals in a variety of environments. With fish, for example, you can learn a certain amount by dissecting them, but you won't know how they move and feed without studying them in water. And you won't learn about their behaviour with other fish and predators unless you observe them in a realistic environment. Even then, you will not get to know about them fully unless you become a total observer of them.

So it is in medicine. In order to help someone you need to know as much as possible about their condition, their symptoms and the things that make their symptoms better or worse. And, ideally, you want to know about their habits, their diet, their desires, their fears, their relationships and so on. That might seem like a tall order, but if you can build up such a picture of the sufferer, then you can see how a condition is truly affecting them throughout all levels of their life.

And this is what you need to do in order to help yourself manage a condition in the most effective way that you can. This model enables the individual to build a picture of their life and the way that the different spheres of their life interact in a cyclical manner.

There are six levels or spheres of life that we need to consider:

- *Body* – what symptoms you have, e.g. pain, stiffness, tiredness.

- *Emotions* – how you feel, e.g. anxious, sad, depressed, angry or jealous of others.

- *Mind* – the type of thoughts you have, e.g. pessimistic thoughts, negative thoughts, self-defeating thoughts.

- *Behaviour* – how it makes you behave, e.g. isolating yourself by avoiding things or people. Or by developing habits, e.g. smoking, drinking, becoming inactive.

- *Lifestyle* – how it affects your ability to do things, your relationships, and also how events in your life impact on you.

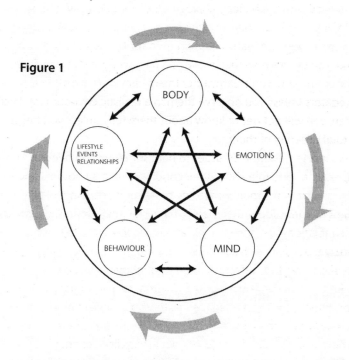

Figure 1

Now take a look at Figure 1. You will see the five spheres starting with the Body sphere at the top. If you follow it clockwise you will see that it follows the order above – body, emotions, mind, behaviour, and lifestyle. And note the outer circle that encloses the whole structure. This represents the individual's whole self, their life. In other words, the five spheres all make up part of the individual's experience of life.

Notice that inside the outer ring of arrows there are double-headed arrows between the spheres. The outer arrows represent the general progression, the life cycle, because the order represents the way that a physical condition will tend to impact on a person.

That is, physical symptoms make the individual aware that something is wrong in the body. This can induce an emotional response, which could be anxiety, anger, resentment or fear. This response alters the way that you think and the type of thoughts that you have. This may make you take a particular action or behave in a way: to reach for a drink, take a tablet or go to bed until it goes away. Your actions or behaviours may affect your lifestyle, stopping you doing things, which may affect relationships and work. And all of that can set the cycle off again.

The inner arrows show that every sphere impacts on every single other one. For example, a pain impacts on all spheres of your life. On the other hand, the inner arrows give you the opportunity to use any of the other spheres to reduce the pain or to deal better with it.

And with depression, you can do exactly the same. It is felt in the emotional sphere. It makes you think in a particular way, which makes you tend to act in a particular way and it will impact on your life style. You may or may not feel physical symptoms. Looking at the inner arrows you can see that there are lots of potential ways that, by improving one sphere, you can affect the depression. In realising this you can immediately start to reduce the feeling of hopelessness that tends to go hand-in-hand with depression. So too can you see that you are not helpless; there are all those potential strategies that can help.

Use the Life Cycle to sketch out your life

This is a useful exercise. Get a notebook and make it your Life Cycle diary. Draw the five spheres and label them. Draw all of the arrows as in the diagram. Do it deliberately, carefully, because you are crafting it. It is your Life Cycle and it deserves to look artistic. Take pride in it. Realise also that it is a dynamic thing that you are going to be able to change. Indeed, as you fill up the notebook, which you should do gradually, on a weekly basis, you will see the changes.

So, after the page with the Life Cycle, allocate two facing pages to each sphere. Make an entry on each one. That is, with 'body', just jot down any physical feelings that you have. It may be 'fatigue', or 'palpitations' or 'sore throat' – whatever you are aware of. With 'emotions' it will probably be depression, but try to add words or notes that describe it better. What are you feeling? For 'mind', write down the main thoughts that you have throughout the day. (I find it often helps if you put them in inverted commas, because if you formulate your thought as you would actually say it, you have to mentally process it into language. The inverted commas indicate the exact thought that you had at the time of writing it. This will be useful when you later review it.) And so on to complete the cycle.

You will soon see that some sort of a pattern manifests itself to you. You may feel that it would work better if you score every entry, for example on a scale from −5 to +5, where zero is a neutral score. Thus a pain can be a negative score (with −5 being the worst pain imaginable), whereas a happy feeling is a positive one (with +5 being utter delight). That way you can produce a number for each sphere. The emotion sphere and the mind sphere will probably initially have marked negative scores.

Other people are more visual. They may prefer to use the cycle itself to enter their notes. That way you can make some spheres larger than others. The emotions will probably be very large as will the mind sphere. But as you progress with it, over weeks you should be able to reduce the size of them all to happy, contented, equal spheres, not dominated by the emotions.

By using the other spheres you potentially can use any one or all of them to reduce the weight of any single sphere, which in depression is of course the emotion sphere. You can focus on the body, or on the mind, on the lifestyle or on your actions or behaviour. You will see that you can keep yourself on an even keel.

So now, let us look at the individual spheres.

The sphere of emotion

People who are depressed will probably have had other people tell them to cheer up, or pull their socks up. They will probably have tried telling themselves to do this. They may have gone through a sort of balance sheet in their heads, ticking off all the positives in their life in an attempt to show that they have no need to feel down. Yet it doesn't seem to help. You can't just cheer up. You can't just tell depression to go. Something has to be done to make this happen.

Let me give you an analogy. If you are feeling nervous and fearful with butterflies in your stomach and a rapid heartbeat, you can't say 'heart, slow down' or 'tummy, settle down'. The reason is that these are physiological changes and you can't alter them by just giving an order. You have to induce a reaction that will result in them being settled. The reaction that you need to use is a relaxation response.

There is a technique called progressive muscle relaxation, which is actually very good at producing this relaxation response, and I describe it in the section on the body sphere (p. 172). It is a simple technique that many people with anxiety and depression find useful, and is a good example of the way that one sphere can affect another.

And if it makes one feel more relaxed, then it automatically affects the other spheres as well.

Of course, the emotion sphere that you make notes about, or which you fill up like a balloon if you choose the visual approach, may not simply have the word 'depression' in it. There may be other emotions like guilt, hate, irritability, and hopelessness. Sometimes you need to focus on individual key features like those, which will also have an effect on reducing the weight of the emotion sphere. For example, if you hold a grudge or a hatred of someone, then you might focus on that and attempt to dispel it by trying to forgive.

The sphere of the mind

This is probably the most important sphere, yet it is not the only one to focus on. I firmly believe that you need to consider all of the spheres and get them working for you. Yet the way that you think is of huge relevance because thoughts arise from the emotions, emotions arise from thought patterns, and thoughts and emotions affect and are affected by the other life spheres.

Thoughts arise from the emotions

The sort of thoughts that you have is in part determined by the emotion that you are feeling. If you wake up in the morning and you feel happy, then the train of thought you have is liable to go in a different direction from the one that you will have if you are fearful, guilty, angry or sad.

The emotions do not just turn off by telling them to change. You have to make them change, and one of the most effective ways is by thinking.

Now that is not at all easy, I admit. The person who is depressed is probably trying to do that all the time, but not really succeeding. People who are depressed or who have experienced depression often talk about the constant battle or the constant struggle with their mood and their depression. They may be able to cope with it after a fashion, yet it is an unpleasant experience and a continual uphill battle.

The problem here is that the negative thinking that arises simply reinforces the negative emotion.

Emotions arise from thought patterns

This is extremely important to understand. People who experience depression do not think in the same way as people who never get depressed. They seem to have depressive thinking. This they need to get out of and learn to think positively.

Dr Aaron Beck, one of the originators of Cognitive Therapy, observed that depressive thinking comes about because of the cognitive triad. This is a view that depression-prone people have of themselves, the world and the future.

- Personal view – they have a poor image of themselves as individuals, they feel unworthy, inadequate and they have to make excuses for themselves.

- World view – they can only see the negative side of things, especially in relation to themselves. They will only see what they have done wrong, not what they did well, and they will take any criticism to heart.

- Future – this is only bleak and gloomy. In part, this relates to their feeling of personal inadequacy. Everything that can go wrong will go wrong and it is perceived as their fault.

None of this is at all conscious. It happens automatically, but it can be changed – it will just take time.

Thoughts and emotions affect and are affected by the other life spheres

This is also fundamental. If you are feeling sad and depressed it can make you feel worthless and unattractive. The inevitable consequence is to withdraw and isolate oneself from situations where that feeling might be overwhelming. In other words, the emotion induces and reinforces the thought that you are less than worthy. The behaviour you adopt is to hide away and withdraw. But there are ways to tackle this.

Take away that fear of exposing yourself. That fear is unconscious and when you do something that removes it, the emotion is no longer being reinforced, and so you weaken the depression.

You could do something different in the behaviour sphere, by adopting a different habit. Or in the lifestyle sphere, by joining a club, or meeting relatives and friends more often. Or do something physical in the body sphere, like taking up a new exercise or sport. The attention that you have to give this new activity will reduce the attention that you give to the emotions or thought spheres.

Cultivate optimism

Optimists tend not to get as depressed as pessimists. Pessimists tend to have a lot of negative automatic thought. Let me give you four examples of such negative thought.

Filtering – is where the individual filters out all the positives and sees only the negative. For example, despite a good day at work, they focus on the single error.

Personalisation – whenever something goes wrong they automatically assume it is their fault.

Catastrophising – they extrapolate all situations to the worst scenario, usually finding a reason for not doing something to prevent a supposed humiliation risk.

Polarisation – they see everything as two poles, good or bad, black or white, with nothing between.

To think positively, you have to monitor your self-talk and try to alter the negativity. For example, instead of thinking, 'I can't do it because I have never done it before', try thinking, 'it's an opportunity to learn'. Or instead of 'there is no way this will work for me', try 'let me try to make this work'. Do not accept the false belief that because something happened to you once it will always happen to you. That actually is not logical. You need to expect it not to happen. Start looking on the bright side and expect good things to occur.

Cultivate mindfulness

This really is helpful, and is the essence of Mindfulness-Based Cognitive Therapy, which we considered in Chapter 8. You will recall that it is derived from Mindfulness-Based Stress Reduction and is advocated as a course of eight weeks in order to help people between depression episodes to stay well. It seems to be successful in reducing relapses by around 50 per cent.

Cultivating mindfulness is a way to combat depressive thinking.

For example, pick any activity of normal life, such as drinking a cup of tea or coffee. If one is depressed it probably gives little pleasure, since the mind is not involved in the act of drinking, but is off somewhere else, following a train of thought that is reinforcing the negative emotion. Mindfulness would make you focus on the cup of tea, the way that it was produced, made, the taste, the temperature, the feeling that it induces.

The various tea ceremonies around the world do just this. In China, Korea and Japan there are quite elaborate ceremonies that demand that one focuses on the joy, the pleasure and the harmony of the drinking experience and nature itself. You will see in Chapter 15 that depression rates are very low in Japan; this is attributed to the diet, yet it may be that mindfulness is also a large part of the process.

So, cultivating mindfulness, focusing on the activity in hand rather than allowing the mind to wander into fruitless negativity, is one of the keys.

You should try this throughout the whole day. When driving, rather than allowing the mind to wander to other matters, which it does with most people, focus on the skill of driving. Regrasp the pleasure that you obtained when you first learned to drive. Focus on the comfort of the seat, the pleasantness of the world around you. What you are doing is disengaging the autopilot that leads to depression.

The sphere of behaviour

This is all to do with your actions and habits. Depressive thinking so often leads to depressive actions, which reinforce the feelings of poor self-esteem and the depression itself.

So, if you feel down don't reach for cigarettes, a glass of wine or bottle of beer. Don't order a helping of junk food, but think, what else can you do?

Change habits and change habitat is a good place to start. Think of a place where you permit yourself to lapse into depressive habits. Then change that habitat to a place where it would not be appropriate to carry out the habit. It's rather like stopping smoking: instead of going outside with a packet of cigarettes, change the habitat to somewhere like the kitchen and make a pot of soup or bake a cake. Stay inside in the warmth and revel in the fact that you no longer smell of stale tobacco.

So change the things that you do, focus on them in a mindful way, enjoying the moment, disengaging the autopilot that allows you to punish yourself with negative thinking. Instead of allowing yourself the luxury of feeling depressed, think positively, do things positively and focus on the joy of the moment. Little by little, piece-by-piece you will change that feeling of depression.

The sphere of lifestyle

Friends, family, work; they all have their pluses and minuses. In depression the negatives are all that one sees. Yet with mindfulness and optimistic thinking, you can change all that. Revel in the family. Enjoy being with friends. Take up new activities. Learn a language, take up yoga or meditation, start writing poetry or a novel.

Do different things to get yourself out of the rut, however comfortable that rut may be – and as long as you are depressed, it won't actually be all that comfortable anyway.

The sphere of body

This involves body awareness. Be aware of the positive attributes of the body. Even if you are aware of physical symptoms or if you suffer a physical condition, there are still things about your body that you can enjoy. You need to be comfortable in your own skin. You need to enjoy being you.

If you feel less fit than you think you should be, then do some exercise and address your diet. We will look at this in the following chapters on diet and exercise.

Progressive Muscle Relaxation

This is a technique that is often used in hypnotherapy in order to deepen a state of relaxation. There is no great mystery about it and I recommend it to you as a way to relax.

Sit back in an easy chair or lie down somewhere that you will not be disturbed by the phone or other interruptions. Take your shoes off. Close your eyes and tell yourself that you are going to relax all of your muscles. Tell yourself that as your muscles relax they will become less uncomfortable (using the word 'uncomfortable' rather than 'painful' induces a physiological effect which makes you experience a real relaxation response).

Now clench your fists tightly for a count of seven. As you do this focus your attention on the tightness in the hands, feeling it increase as you count up. Then suddenly let it go, and tell yourself that instead of tension there is now increasing relaxation in those muscles of the hand, and they will get even more relaxed as you count to fifteen.

Now clench your fists and this time also tense the muscles of your feet by trying to clench the toes. Do this for a count of seven, exactly as before. Then release the tension suddenly and let the relaxation deepen for a count of fifteen.

Now do it by clenching all of the muscles of your arms and of your legs, in exactly the same way. Tense for seven and relax for fifteen.

Then tense all of the muscles of all your limbs, clench the buttocks together and tense the stomach muscles and your neck and face muscles. Screw your eyes tightly closed as you count to seven, and then release suddenly and relax for fifteen.

Then tell yourself that your muscles are now going to relax totally and that they will continue to relax and will feel more comfortable when you stop. Now imagine that a wave of relaxation is moving all the way up over your body from your feet, up your legs, up your back and chest to your neck. Let that feeling pass down both arms and up your neck to your head, relaxing all of the muscles as it moves up over the top of your head and down over your face.

Tell yourself that you will enjoy that for a minute or so and if you fall asleep, that's all well and good. But after the time is up just tell yourself that your muscles feel good and they feel continue to feel better, and that they will feel better each time that you do this.

It is as simple as that. And the thing is, the muscles will develop a memory and they will get less uncomfortable over time. Just make it something that you do every day.

Putting it all together

I said that this was not rocket science, yet it is a practical model that people do find useful to at least begin to address their depression and stay well. Get a notebook, do the exercises that I mentioned, practise mindfulness, start to become an optimist, and change habits and habitats.

The model is not intended as a sort of substitute for conventional care. It is simply a means of looking at the different spheres of your life to see how you can introduce self-help. It is also to be used to see how talking therapies, medication that may have been prescribed or other strategies can be charted so that you can assess how you are doing, and how they dovetail with the other areas of your life.

KEY POINTS

- Be aware of the cognitive triad of depressive thinking – personal view, world view, future view. You can change them.
- Mindfulness is the way to focus on the moment, the instant, the activity and seek pleasure and joy in it.
- Optimists enjoy life, pessimists are more liable to depression. Be an optimist.
- Working on the Life Cycle can give you a model to improve the sphere of emotion.

Chapter 15

A healthy diet

Let food be thy medicine and medicine be thy food.

Hippocrates (460–370 BC), the father of medicine

Diet and depression is a cloudy area

There is an old adage that 'you are what you eat'. And there is yet another that says 'one man's meat is another man's poison'. I like these old aphorisms, as you may have gathered from my use of a quote at the start of each chapter. I have tried to make each one appropriate for the subject of the chapter. I think that they actually serve a purpose, for they implant a message in the mind of the reader. And generally, I think they are helpful messages.

Let us take the above quote from Hippocrates, the father of medicine. He was a physician working in classical Greece. He raised the practice of medicine from a mixture of religion, ritual and magic to an actual science. He firmly believed that nutrition was important in the treatment of most cases of illness. He even talked about using the herb that is known to us as St John's wort for melancholia and other conditions. He suggested that it should be taken as food. And after over two millennia, we know that it is a herb that actually helps a lot of people with depression.

The two adages that I mentioned are also of interest. Firstly, we actually are what we eat, since we digest and absorb our food in order to use the various nutrients for energy, to give us the building blocks for our internal chemistry and to build our tissues. Good food should keep us well; by that line of reasoning, 'bad' food may make us less well or unwell.

Yet it is also the case that some people cannot tolerate the foods that others can. Some people may take foods that make them unwell or which make them feel depressed, but which other people can eat without any adverse effect.

There may seem to be some contradiction in the adages. Well, that is understandable, because they are simply rules of thumb, little snippets that may have a practical benefit. You cannot encapsulate all of the best advice about diet in a line or two, after all.

Or can you? In fact, I think that one can draw some simple conclusions about nutrition and depression that may help a lot of people. I have deliberately chosen that quote and those two adages to show that the whole issue of nutrition is cloudy, just as the question about whether food can help depression is cloudy. Yet I do want to arrive at a few simple guidelines. To get there, I want to look at three simple areas that we can look at practically to help ease depression:

- Foods that may cause depression

- Foods that may help depression

- Dietary discipline or chaos.

Avoid depressive foods

It has often been observed that people who become depressed don't seem to eat a balanced diet. For some, it seems that the diet may deteriorate once they have become depressed, yet others have a poor diet to begin with. The question as to whether a 'poor' or 'bad' diet can cause depression is obviously of great importance, since unipolar depression is actually one of the leading causes of disability-adjusted years lost within developed countries.[12] (This is a measure of the burden that diseases impose on a country. It was developed by Harvard University and is used by the World Health Organisation for research into health.)

Depression affects 150 million people worldwide, but rates vary immensely country by country. The incidence can be 60 times greater in some countries than in others. The UK and the USA have rates at the upper ends, compared with Korea and Japan where it is very low. Studies have suggested that countries that have seen a decline in, for example, fish eating have noticed a rise in the rate of depression. This seems to be in line with the increasing consumption of fast food and so-called junk food.

This issue was looked at in a study from Spain in 2012, to see whether people's consumption of fast foods and baked goods, such as pies and pastries, could be associated with depression. They found a significant link.

The study was carried out by a research team from the University of Las Palmas in Gran Canaria and the University of Navarra, led by Dr Almudena Sánchez-Villegas. It was funded by the Spanish Government's Carlos III Institute of Health, and it was published in the journal *Public Health Nutrition*.[13] They looked at 9,000 people who had been recruited to the SUN study (Seguimiento Universidad de Navarra), which is a long-running cohort study of university graduates. It continuously collects new graduates as recruits and follows them up over several years using questionnaires. None of the 9,000 had any previous history of depression.

The study was very useful in establishing what people were eating before the study started, rather than just looking at how their diet may have changed if they became depressed. They showed that people who consumed the most fast food – pies, pizzas and pastries – were 37 per cent more likely to become depressed over six years than people with the lowest consumption of these types of food.

More than that, they were actually able to demonstrate a dose-response. This means that the more you eat, the greater the risk.

It may be the trans-fats

So what could it be that causes the problem? Is it that there is something in fast food or junk food that isn't in other diets? Or could eating such food mean you are deficient in things that are present in other diets?

Both are likely, I think.

Another piece of research from the SUN study, this time in 2011, implies that the trans-fats are the problem.[14] In looking at over 12,000 SUN project volunteers they found that after six years 657 had developed depression. Of those depressed volunteers, those with the highest consumption of trans-fats had a 48 per cent increase in the risk of depression compared to those with the lowest levels.

Trans-fats are produced when oils have been hydrogenated. This allows them to have a longer shelf life. You will find them in many packaged foods, pastries, fast foods, French fries and microwavable popcorn.

Again, the problem seems to be that they promote inflammation, which I will return to further on because I think it is a possible factor in depression.

It could be the lack of certain nutrients

Fast foods tend to have more salt than is desirable, since too much may take the sodium content above the recommended daily intake. Whether sodium is in any way involved with depression, we have no real evidence about.

On the other hand, a diet of fast or junk food may well be deficient in dietary fibre and other essential micronutrients like minerals and vitamins that seem to have an effect on mood. If they are the mainstay of one's diet then you could end up with relative deficiency of these important components of the diet. In particular, vitamin B3, B6, folate, B12, and the minerals zinc, magnesium and, as we shall see later, essential fatty acids.

Folate levels are very important. As long ago as 1976 it was established by researchers at King's College Hospital that one-third of the patients who presented with psychiatric conditions, including depression, were deficient in folate.

A study from Finland looked at 2,313 men who were discharged from hospital after a period of depression.[15] They were followed up for 10–15 years. It was found that those with a below-mean intake of folate were far more likely to suffer from recurrent episodes of depression.

Foods that help mood

So what foods can help? Well, studies of the rates of depression have consistently shown that they are lower in Mediterranean countries than they are in Northern European countries. That and the fact that suicide rates in Mediterranean countries are also lower,[16] inevitably pose the question, why?

As mentioned earlier, studies have shown that countries which have reduced their consumption of fish have experienced rising levels of depression. This naturally turns the attention to diet, specifically to the Mediterranean diet. So is there any hard evidence that it is at least protective against depression? Indeed there is, and we return to yet more research from the SUN study, published in the *Archives of Psychiatry* in 2009.[17]

This time the research team, again led by Dr Almudena Sánchez-Villegas, studied 10,094 SUN volunteers over four years and found that those who consumed a classic Mediterranean diet were 30 per cent less likely to develop depression.

Another study from 2009 looked at 3,486 British civil servants over five years and came to exactly the same conclusion. Those who ate a Mediterranean-style diet were 30 per cent less likely to develop depression.[18] They also found that those who ate a processed-food diet had a higher risk.

The Mediterranean diet

The characteristics of the so-called Mediterranean diet are:

- High levels of fruits and vegetables, breads and other cereals, potatoes, beans, nuts, and seeds.

- Olive oil is the only fat allowed.

- Moderate amounts of dairy products, fish, and poultry, but very little red meat.

- Eggs allowed, but no more than four per week and no more than one on any day.

- Wine consumed in moderate amounts—two glasses per day for men, one glass for women.

The fish and the olive oil seem to be two of the most significant features of the diet.

Olive oil seems to be rich in monounsaturated fatty acids. It is suggested that its benefit may be in improving the way that serotonin, the 'happiness neurotransmitter', is bound to its receptors.

A study of nine European countries found that the lowest levels of depression occurred in Spain[19] which, along with Greece, happens to be the two highest consumers of olive oil.[20]

Fish is rich in omega-3 fats, and these seem to be the factors that benefit us most. They certainly seem to have an anti-inflammatory effect.

A SHORT LESSON ABOUT FATS AND OILS

Everyone knows that you must not take too much fat into your system, and yet you hear about the benefits of various types of oils. Understandably, there is a lot of confusion about fats and oils. I shall try to present this as simply as possible.

There are three basic types of fats – saturated, monounsaturated and polyunsaturated.

Saturated fats are found in animal products such as meat, eggs and dairy products. In general, these are considered 'bad' fats, since they have a tendency to push up your cholesterol and also promote inflammation.

Monounsaturated fats are found in various nuts including peanuts, walnuts and almonds, avocados and olive oil. They help to lower cholesterol and are 'good' fats, which can help to reduce inflammation.

Polyunsaturated fats are the best ones, and are found in seafood and fish, corn oil and sunflower oil. They help to lower cholesterol and they are also anti-inflammatory. They are composed of two groups of essential fatty acids, called omega-3 and omega-6.

There are two types of omega-3s, those with long chains and those with short chains. The long chains are mainly found in oily fish. The two main ones are called eicosapentaenoic acid (EPA) and docosahexaenoic acid (DHA). These are anti-inflammatory and they have been found to be good for both arthritis and the heart and seemingly also depression.

Short chain omega-3s are found in foods like soya, flax, pumpkin seeds, walnuts and leafy green vegetables. They can be converted by the body into the long-chain fatty acids that do the most good.

You will find that lots of foods, like spreads, juices and even milk, have added omega-3s. This is good as the average British diet is really quite deficient in omega-3s. Yet the thing is that it is more efficient to get the omega-3s in their natural form, from oily fish, such as salmon, mackerel, sardines. Aim at having two, or even better, three portions a week. But take care if you are prone to gout!

Olive oil, the only oil in the Mediterranean diet, contains no omega-3s. Its main constituent is oleic acid, which belongs to the omega-9s. It is a bit of a mystery, but research is ongoing into its undoubted benefits. It certainly seems to have marked anti-inflammatory effects.

Inflammation

This is the body's response whenever the integrity of the body is breached, by trauma or invasion by microbes. It has been recognised since antiquity, when the Roman encyclopaedist Aulus Cornelius Celsus (25 BC–AD 50) wrote a book entitled *de Medicina*. He was not a doctor himself, but he wrote about the knowledge of medicine and surgery of his times. He describes the four cardinal signs of inflammation as follows: *calor* (warmth), *dolor* (pain), *tumor* (swelling) and *rubor* (heat). These are the same features that every doctor and nurse are taught about to this day.

Inflammation can occur inside the body and can affect any organ. The origin can be the result of trauma, infection or auto-immunity, when the body starts to fight itself. In medicine, we are discovering new things about the way that inflammation may be at the root of many conditions that were previously thought to have no inflammatory component. It is thought that some cases of depression, although not all by any means, could have an inflammation component.

There are various conditions that are definitely inflammatory, which are also associated with depression. Rheumatoid arthritis and various chronic arthritis conditions are examples. It was always assumed that the depression was a secondary psychological effect, since these conditions can be debilitating and it would be understandable that they can make one feel down. Yet, as indicated in the Cytokine Hypothesis in Chapter 4, there is evidence that inflammation can actually be a physical cause in itself for depression.

The Cytokine Hypothesis

From our consideration of the Cytokine Hypothesis and the evidence for it, there certainly seems to be legitimate reasons why diet can be important in both causing and reducing the risk of depression.

Junk food promotes inflammation

As we have seen above, there is clinical evidence from the SUN study that fast food or junk food is associated with increased rates of depression. How does it do this, you may ask?

It seems to do it by virtue of the tendency of junk food to promote inflammation. By junk food I mean 'fast' food with added fat, sugar and salt, and processed foods with lots of additives. The fats used in its preparation include trans fats and saturated fats. These promote inflammation because arachidonic acid, one of the fatty acids found in these fats, is broken down by enzymes into prostaglandins and leukotrienes. These are chemicals that are known to trigger inflammation.

Diets high in sugar have also been associated with increased inflammation, as well as predisposing you to obesity and diabetes. It is worth eliminating high-sugar foods such as fizzy drinks, pastries, pre-sweetened cereals and confectionary. It doesn't mean that you shouldn't have them as treats; just don't have them regularly.

Omega oils are anti-inflammatory

The fact that the omega oils in the Mediterranean diet are anti-inflammatory looks to be another piece in the jigsaw. The Mediterranean diet is basically anti-inflammatory, whereas processed food diets are inflammatory. The fact that the Mediterranean diet is associated with a reduction in risk of inflammation, while the processed diet is associated with an increase in risk, all fits in with the Cytokine Hypothesis.

Dietary chaos

People who become depressed often have irregular eating habits, maybe even quite chaotic ones, sometimes binging on carbohydrates, sometimes missing meals, or eating on the hoof. Our high pressured lifestyles may contribute to that, but basically if you are not able to eat regularly and allow adequate time to digest, then you do not absorb the food as well as you need to.

One of the reasons that fast food outlets do so well is because people are in a hurry, but fast eating is not good for your system. Skipping meals, eating on the move, bolting food down or eating too late are all patterns that tend to lead to problems.

All of your digestive functions are controlled by part of your nervous system, which only operates effectively when you are calm and at rest. When you are up and being busy then it pretty well shuts down so that your muscles get the lion's share of oxygen. This means that the digestion is delayed until later and the food just sits there fermenting. This can lead to bloating, excess gas in the bowel, which causes increased pressure in the bowel. It can also lead to constipation. These disturbances have an effect on the mood.

You should aim to eat at regular times, preferably sitting at a table, having wholesome nutrient-rich, fresh food rather than processed meals with extra fat, salt and sugar. Get out of the habit of having a quick sandwich or worst of all, eating on the go. Regular eating seems associated with more even moods.

Tryptophan

You may have heard that turkey at Christmas is good for people, because it lifts the mood. The reason, it seems, is the tryptophan content.

All of the fowls are rich in tryptophan, with goose at the top of the league table. Next comes duck, and then turkey and chicken with round about the same amounts, pound for pound. Other good sources of tryptophan are milk, cheese, bread and bananas.

Tryptophan is an important amino acid in the diet, because it is used to build serotonin, which is one of the main neurotransmitters within the brain. Unfortunately, the absorption of tryptophan from the diet depends on several factors. For example, if there are lots of other amino acids available for the body to choose from, then there is a sort of competition to see which are taken in. Tryptophan is often not absorbed whereas other amino acids are.

This is quite significant, according to research published in the journal *Brain, Behaviour and Immunity*. Dutch researchers have shown that people with a family history of depression are 50 per cent more likely to feel down if their tryptophan levels fall. Ten per cent of those without such a family history also feel down when their levels fall.

Low levels of tryptophan are liable to occur in people taking high-protein and low-carbohydrate diets, which have become very popular lately. Low levels also occur in those not eating properly through illness, depression, or through various types of fad dieting. Body builders also need to be careful about how they eat, because they can get down in the dumps without realising why. This can be the case if they are taking in lots of amino acids at once, since the tryptophan may not be absorbed. And the same goes for people who are already down; they may create a vicious circle that feeds their depression.

One important point about tryptophan, however, is the fact that to activate it you need to take carbohydrate and Vitamin B6 at the same time. And this is perhaps why turkey with cranberry sauce and red wine literally goes down so well at Christmas, by providing all the carbohydrate you need and the Vitamin B6.

Chapter 16

Exercise and depression

If we could give every individual the right amount of nourishment and exercise, not too little and not too much, we would have found the safest way to health.

Hippocrates (460–370 BC), the father of medicine

The gymnasium spirit

Hippocrates lived during the Classic Age of Greece. This was an era of tremendous advancement in the fields of mathematics, philosophy and medicine. He taught that people should take charge of their own health and should look after and train both the body and the mind.

The gymnasium was an important part of life in Ancient Greece. It was a place where the young would go to train their bodies for games and competitions, but also where they could discuss, learn and have their minds stimulated. It became a place of physical fitness and also became associated with medicine and education. Philosophers gave lectures and held talks and gradually the gymnasium became a place to enhance the health of both the body and the mind.

In Athens there were three great gymnasia: the Academy, the Lyceum and the Cynosarges. Each was dedicated to a deity and each became associated with one of the schools of philosophy. Plato had a school associated with the Academy. Aristotle had one at the Lyceum, and Antisthenes, the founder of the school of cynics, established one at the Cynosarges.

This concept of mind and body training at the gymnasium is an ancient one, and is worth knowing about. Today, we associate the gymnasium with physical exercise. The intellectual and mind-nurturing aspect has been lost, yet study after study demonstrates that exercise does not just help the body, it also helps the mood. Although the gymnasium is no longer associated with a place of learning, yet the value of exercise in helping the mood means that the spirit of the gymnasium lives on.

Exercise and mood

There have been many studies on exercise and mood since the early 1970s. They have generally shown that exercise helps people feel better. For example, in 1976 Folkins studied the effect of physical exercise on men at risk of having a heart attack and compared them with a group of men with the same risk, who remained sedentary.[21] As the exercise group became fitter their moods improved. Other studies on other groups showed a similar result.

Exercise and depression

Whether this change in mood could help people who are depressed is another matter. This has been addressed in several studies. In 2001,

Dr F. Dimeo at the Free University of Berlin looked at this by studying the effect of exercise on twelve people, five men and seven women, who had been diagnosed with major depression.[22] They had on average suffered from depression for nine months. They had a course of aerobic exercise which consisted of walking on a treadmill for 30 minutes a day for ten days. Their depression levels were measured using the Hamilton Rating Scale for Depression. After the course, all of their depression ratings dropped very significantly. The authors concluded that exercise could probably have been as effective as drug treatment in helping mild to moderate depression.

Another study was performed at Duke University in North Carolina, USA, by a team led by J. A. Blumenthal. This looked at 156 patients over the age of 50 who had been diagnosed with major depression.[23] They were randomised into three groups. One group received antidepressants, another group had aerobic exercise only, and a third group had a combination of the two. Quite surprisingly, all three groups improved by the same amount. Exercise was as good as antidepressants, but the combination of the two did not show any additional improvement.

Another very interesting study was published in the *American Journal of Preventive Medicine* in 2005.[24] This study was carried out between 1998 and 2001 with eight patients who had been diagnosed with mild to moderate depression. The researchers looked to see whether the amount of exercise that was done could have a 'dose response'. That is, whether more intense exercise was better than gentle exercise, and whether the time taken was relevant. They found that the ideal dosage was half an hour on six days a week. This seemed to produce a significant reduction in depression score using the Hamilton Rating Scale. Less than that had no more effect than a placebo.

How does exercise help?

The answer is that we do not precisely know, but we do have an idea that it has a beneficial psychological effect and a real physical effect on the way that the brain functions. It exerts its effect on the brain by boosting several types of natural chemicals and various neurotransmitters. We shall focus on three: serotonin – the 'happiness neurotransmitter'; endorphins – the 'runner's high'; and Brain-derived Neurotrophic Factor – a mysterious neurotransmitter.

Serotonin

We have seen throughout this book that when serotonin levels drop, depression seems to occur. The SSRI group of antidepressants helps to keep the serotonin level up, which improves depression.

Although serotonin affects the brain, over 75 per cent of the serotonin in the body is found in cells in the gut. A study published in *Neuropsychopharmacology* suggests that there are two ways in which exercise increases brain levels of serotonin. One way is by increased motor activity, the firing rates of serotonin neurons are increased. That is, it somehow stimulates the brain cells to release more serotonin. Secondly, regular exercise increases the level of tryptophan in the brain. This is an amino acid that is used to manufacture serotonin.

Endorphins

The endorphins are the body's natural painkillers. They are released when you exercise and are well known for producing the 'runner's high', a sense of euphoria after a good run. They are also released when one has acupuncture.

The endorphin response to exercise increases with frequency of exercising. Indeed, it may seem to many people that they end up having to exercise because they get addicted to it. Well, it is not really an addiction, but they may very well like the feeling that they get, as well as enjoying the psychological effect of staying fit.

The exercise does not have to be extreme; even gentle exercise will boost endorphins.

Brain-derived Neurotrophic Factor

This is a neurotrophin, a protein that is involved in the development and functioning of neurons (nerve cells). It is found in the brain, in particular in areas called the hippocampus, brain cortex and basal forebrain.

BDNF levels have been found to be depleted in people with depression.[25] It is also reduced in other conditions, including obsessive–compulsive disorder, schizophrenia, anorexia nervosa and dementia. Its exact role in depression is unclear, yet it seems that exercise, which increases BDNF, may help because this is one of the things that it boosts.

KEY POINTS

- NICE recommend group-based exercise for mild-to-moderate depression.

Finding the right exercise for you

Any exercise is good for you. The thing is to choose an activity that is enjoyable and not a chore. Exercise does not have to be a sport; it can be gardening, housework, or walking a dog. It doesn't have to be competitive, but if competition helps your mood, then choose a competitive sport. That can vary from field sports, if appropriate for your age and fitness, to less vigorous ones, like golf and bowling. Think also about dance classes, ranging from salsa to ballroom or even ballet. And it is never too late to start. Many dance schools offer novice classes for all ages.

It is a good idea to discuss exercise with your GP before you start. It is sensible to know that your blood pressure is at a healthy level and that you are not going to harm yourself by taking up something that is too much for you.

Joining a gym or a sports club is also a good idea, because the social element can be important in helping to elevate the mood. Most gyms offer personal trainers, who can work with you to organise your fitness programme.

KEY POINTS

- Adults 19–64 should be doing 150 minutes of exercise a week.
- Adults over 65 should be aiming at 75 minutes of exercise a week.
- All age groups benefit from exercising.

How often you do the exercise depends upon the pressures on your week, but three sessions a week would be adequate. My own advice is to do half an hour six days a week and a day off. It does not take long before you start to feel better when exercising. One study by Hansen and Stevens[26] showed that you actually start to feel better after ten minutes and then continue to feel better up to another 20 minutes. Half an hour therefore seems adequate.

Many GP practices offer advice about exercise and may have walking groups, often organised by the attached health visitor, that meet so many days a week in order to walk routes in the locality. This is helpful for people suffering from depression, bereavement and anxiety. It may also be possible to have supervised exercise for a number of sessions, 'prescribed' on the NHS.

A study published in *Women & Health* looked at how long the beneficial effects of exercise were felt.[27] R. E. Lee and co-researchers found that the beneficial effect on mood of walking daily for seven days a week for seven weeks lasted for five months after the study finished.

The type of exercise doesn't have to be just one activity; there is benefit in varying it, for example by cycling one day, swimming another, hitting golf balls on another, and walking on a couple of days. Variation is good.

Chapter 17

Music, dance and other strategies

Music produces a kind of pleasure which human nature cannot do without.   Confucius (551–479 BC), Chinese philosopher

Music has charms to soothe a savage beast.
             William Congreve (1670–1729), English dramatist and poet

The creative arts

There are various art therapies which may help people with depression. In this context, they are not merely practising an art form as a hobby, but actually using the art form in a therapeutic manner under the guidance of a trained therapist.

These therapies are said to be particularly helpful if you have issues about discussing your feelings. Thus, interpreting your feelings in art, music or dance may be beneficial.

The art therapies include music therapy, dance therapy, art therapy, dramatherapy and voice movement therapy, amongst others.

Music soothes depression

The use of music to help melancholia was advocated in 1621 by Richard Burton in his classic book *The Anatomy of Melancholy*. People have enjoyed music ever since the first musical instruments were made and it is generally accepted that it is good for lifting the spirits. It is also good to know that research has backed this up, especially in its ability to help depression.

A small trial of music therapy was carried out by researchers in Finland and Norway in 2011, which was published in the *British Journal of Psychiatry*.[28] The researchers looked at 79 patients aged 18–50 with diagnosed depression. They were randomised into two groups; the first group received individual music therapy with two sessions a week for ten weeks, in combination with their standard treatment with antidepressants and psychotherapy. The music therapy consisted of having instruction by a music therapist with either a percussion instrument or an acoustic djembe drum. The other group only received standard treatment.

At the end of the trial, then after three months and after six months, clinical ratings for anxiety and depression were taken for each member of each group. The music group scored significantly higher improvements in depression rating. The music group had a 50 per cent reduction, compared to a 22 per cent reduction in the group with standard treatment alone. The research suggests that music therapy has a potentially highly beneficial effect in the treatment of depression. More research needs to be done, however, to determine whether the effects are long term.

A Cochrane analysis of music therapy for depression looked at five studies of music therapy used in addition to standard care and found that four of the five showed greater reduction in symptoms than the standard treatment alone. (The Cochrane Collaboration was established in 1993 and is an independent international network that provides practitioners, consumers and health policy makers with evidence-based research.)

This does not mean that music on its own can improve depression, but it is certainly suggestive that having musical instrument instruction can help.

Singing also is good for lifting the spirits and people who sing in choirs testify that they feel better as a result of the discipline, the camaraderie and the simple joy of singing.

Composing your own song may be helpful in that the creative process may bring things to the front of the mind. If you write it down you may find that your expressive block improves and you may then be better able to talk about your feelings.

Dance therapy

Dance therapy, also called dance movement therapy, is used to help the individual to express themselves through dance and movement. It is based on the theory that people tend to hold their bodies in a manner that mirrors their feelings. Dance therapy encourages the person to allow movement and dance to express their feelings in a creative manner. The whole aim is to get mind and body working together. This can be done individually with a dance therapist or in a group.

Art therapy

I worked in a small psychiatric unit before I became a General Practitioner. It was a therapeutic community house with its own art therapist. I used to envy her, since her working day revolved around painting, pottery, sculpture and story-telling. It looked fun and the patients really seemed to enjoy doing it.

But, as with music and dance therapy, there is more to it than that. She was using the arts to help people to get in touch with their feelings and to express them through the different media. The artwork that they produced was often astonishing. Indeed, people who had never touched a paintbrush since their schooldays often discovered a talent as they tapped into their emotions. And in expressing them, some of our depressed patients found that they were actively making themselves feel better. Ever since then, I have encouraged people to use the arts to help themselves.

Telling a story is another useful form of art therapy. It doesn't need to be the story of how they arrived at the stage they are at, but it is a useful means of allowing buried emotions and memories and associations to come out.

The thing is that you do not have to worry about being good at any of these arts. Just doing them is therapeutic, and trusting in the therapy will help.

Dramatherapy

This is another therapy that is worth considering. Dramatherapy may be available individually or in a group. Dramatherapists are skilled at finding the best medium for people to work in. No previous experience in acting or theatre is needed.

Again, all sorts of techniques are used, including puppetry, masks, improvisations and the use of myths, stories and plays. It can help you learn how to take control of your life and feel what it is like to say no or to be assertive.

It can be very useful to explore issues that may have had a large part to play in someone's depression, and by using dramatherapy techniques the individual may find useful ways of addressing painful issues.

Voice movement therapy (VMT)

This therapy makes a lot of sense. Using the voice to communicate has two aspects: the words that you say – which reflect the thoughts that you have, and the way that you say them – the tones and qualities of the voice reflect the emotions.

A VMT practitioner can work individually or in a group. Like all of the other therapies they work with people with all sorts of issues, including depression.

The client may be helped to find their voice, to help them to communicate by speech and by song, all aiming to promote self-expression, and increase self-confidence and self-esteem, which are all very important if one is depressed.

Finding therapists

Your GP may be able to advise you about local therapists. Otherwise check the organisations listed at the end of the book.

Complementary medicine

For mild depression, many people opt for various complementary therapies and find them to be valuable.

Acupuncture

This is treatment of specific acupuncture points with needles. There are two types of acupuncture practised in the UK: Traditional Chinese Medicine acupuncture based on Traditional Chinese Medicine theory about the flow of energy along meridians, and Western Medical Acupuncture based on Western physiology and clinical medicine. In the treatment of depression, however, the treatment given would be broadly similar.

Homoeopathy

Homoeopathy is a gentle form of medicine based on the 'simile principle'. The word was coined by Dr Samuel Hahnemann (1755–1843) from the Greek words *homoios*, meaning similar or like, and *pathos*, meaning suffering. Essentially, this means that it is a therapeutic method using preparations of substances whose effects, when administered to healthy subjects, correspond to the manifestations of the disorder (the symptoms, clinical signs and pathological states) in the patient. It is a system that is practised across the world. Most of the remedies, of which there are in excess of 4,000, are referred to by their Latin names.

Treatment is very much tailor-made to the patient. With depression, ten patients could well each need a different remedy tailored to their symptom pattern. This is the great difficulty about doing research on this discipline, since there is no such thing as a homoeopathic painkiller or a homoeopathic anti-inflammatory tablet or homoeopathic antidepressant. The remedy treats the person, not a specific symptom or condition.

To get the most out of this method it is probably as well to see a qualified homoeopath. At a consultation, the homoeopathic practitioner will go through all of your symptoms, focusing on how you feel, and going into the things that make symptoms better or worse.

Reflexology

This is a therapy that involves a specific type of massage and manipulation of various reflex areas on the hands and feet. The theory is that points on the feet are reflexly associated with other parts of the body and that massaging those points will have a beneficial effect on the part it is related to. A reflexology treatment is done on all areas of both feet, aiming to treat the whole person, including the brain and the mind. Patients feel that a top-up with reflexology can keep their mood at a level they can cope with.

Reiki

Practitioners call this an energy type of healing. The word is Japanese and means Universal Life Energy. It was developed in Japan by Dr Mikao Isui. Practitioners claim that it is an energy healing system, based on the belief that thoughts have the power to direct energy. Practitioners aim to tune into energy flow through the person to determine imbalances in that flow. The treatment is done lying down with the clothes on. The practitioner places hands non-intrusively in various positions over the body and the patient is encouraged to use visualisation techniques. Some patients experience a marked lifting of the mood.

Yoga

There are different styles of yoga. Some (such as Ananda and Kundalini yoga) are more meditational and spiritual, while others (such as Hatha yoga and Iyengar yoga) are more physical and aim to teach you how to stretch, relax and get into particular postures.

In 2007, researchers from Boston University School of Medicine led by Dr Chris Streeter, looked at changes in levels of a particular neurotransmitter called GABA (gamma-aminobutyric acid – another of the neurotransmitters that is thought to be involved in the runaway thoughts that occur in people who get depressed or anxious) in the brains of experienced yoga practitioners.[29] They compared them before and after they had done a 60-minute yoga practice and compared them to the levels of a control group who had read for an hour. The yoga group had a 27 per cent increase in their levels, whereas no change was found in the readers. They concluded that yoga could be beneficial for people with anxiety and depression who may have low levels of GABA.

In 2010, another study was performed in Boston, again led by Dr Streeter.[30] The researchers found that three sessions of yoga a week boosted depressed patients' levels of GABA, in direct correlation with improvement in their depression.

Conclusion

There is always someone or something that can help.

Depression can seem unfathomable when you are in the midst of an episode. Although ostensibly everything may be going well in your life, yet this black mantle of despair may descend and life may seem to have lost its joy, its sparkle and even its purpose. But it need not be like that. There is always something that can help.

In this book I have tried to take you on a journey through the many theories about depression, and looked at some of the strategies and treatments that are available. If you are depressed there is no need, and indeed no point, in suffering in silence with it. There are excellent treatments available and most people do respond to them and do come out of their depression. It is often a matter of finding out what is the right treatment for you.

But the main thing is to recognise that you need help. Above all else, that is my main purpose in writing this book. You then only have to take the step to begin your journey to feel well again.

I leave you with one final quote:

A journey of a thousand miles begins with a single step.

Lao Tzu (604–531 BC), Chinese philosopher, *The Way of Lao Tzu*

Glossary

acupuncture – a treatment using dry needles to stimulate acupuncture points.

antidepressant – a drug that combats depression.

anticoagulant – a drug that stops the blood from clotting.

anticonvulsant – a drug that prevents epileptic convulsions.

anxiolytic – a drug used to alleviate anxiety.

art therapy – one of the creative arts used in a psychotherapeutic manner.

aspirin – an anti-inflammatory drug.

augmentation – the use of one drug to work with another to produce an enhanced effect.

baby blues – lowness of mood after birth, experienced by two-thirds of women. It starts on day 3 or 4 and clears up spontaneously by day 10.

BDNF or Brain-derived Neurotrophic Factor – a protein that is involved in the development and functioning of neurons (nerve cells).

bipolar disorder – when there are mood swings and both mania and depressed mood.

CBT or Cognitive Behavioural Therapy – one of the talking therapies, working on the basis that the person has learned to think in a particular way.

CMHT – the community mental health team.

cognitive triad – a view that depression prone people have to view themselves, the world and the future. First coined by Aaron Beck.

counselling – one of the talking therapies.

couple therapies – one of the talking therapies.

cytokine – small protein molecules found in the brain and central nervous system which are involved in cell-signalling.

Cytokine Hypothesis – a theory about depression, linking it with underlying inflammation.

delusion – a false fixed belief that is impervious to reason; a feature of a psychotic illness.

depression – persistent lowness of mood.

Diogenes syndrome – a condition of the elderly where the individual hoards rubbish and becomes neglectful of themselves.

double depression – when dysthymic individuals sink into a deep depression, then revert to their normal dysthymic state.

dopamine – one of the neurotransmitters.

DIT or Dynamic Interpersonal Therapy – one of the talking therapies.

The Doctrine of Humors – the theory that dominated medical thought for most of the first two millenia which stated that there were four fundamental humors or body fluids, which determined the state of health of the individual.

dramatherapy – one of the creative arts used in a psychotherapeutic manner.

dysthymia – permanently flattened mood.

ECG or electrocardiogram – a test to measure the electrical activity of the heart.

ECT or electro-convulsive therapy – a treatment involving the passage of electricity through the brain.

emotion – a feeling, e.g. anger.

endorphin – the body's natural painkillers, associated with 'runner's high'.

GABA or gamma-aminobutyric acid – one of the neurotransmitters.

grief – the emotion cased by loss of something or of someone.

hallucination – a perception that something is real when it has no stimulus, but is purely a product of the mind. Can be visual (seeing things) or auditory (hearing voices).

hypochondriasis – fixation with illness, relating it to oneself.

iatrogenic – an illness resulting from drug treatment or other medical treatment.

hypnotherapy – the use of the hypnotic trance to achieve a therapeutic purpose.

ITP or Interpersonal Psychotherapy – one of the talking therapies.

Life Cycle – a self-help model.

Jungian analysis – one of the talking therapies based on the work of Carl Jung.

logotherapy – one of the talking therapies based on the work of Viktor Frankl.

mania – a mood swing into a high state of energy, hilarity, with pressure of thought and pressure of speech.

MBCT or Mindfulness-Based Cognitive Therapy – one of the talking therapies designed to prevent or reduce the severity of depression relapses.

Mindfulness – paying attention to the present moment, deliberately, without judgement.

monoamine – natural messenger chemicals that act as neurotransmitters.

Monoamine Hypothesis – one of the theories of depression, which postulates that depression is caused by a depletion of monoamine neurotransmitters in the nervous system.

music therapy – one of the creative arts used in a psychotherapeutic manner.

neuron – a nerve cell.

neurosis – one of the older classifications of mental disorder.

NLP or Neuro Linguistic Programming – a talking therapy looking at the way one thinks (neuro), how one communicates (linguistic) and how you can teach (programming) the mind to think, communicate and perform more successfully.

neurotransmitter – a natural messenger chemical that is involved in the transmission of signals along nerves and between brain cells.

NICE or National Institute for Health and Care Excellence – an advisory body on all treatments, funded by the Department of Health.

optimism – a positive outlook.

paradoxical intention – one of the treatment techniques used in logotherapy.

paranoia – the misbelief that people are talking about or are conspiring against one.

paraphrenia – a psychotic illness also known as psychosis in the elderly, characterised by paranoid thoughts.

parasuicide – an attempt at suicide, usually by overdosing on drugs.

pessimism – a negative outlook.

postnatal depression (PND) – a depressive illness after giving birth.

postpartum psychosis – a serious psychotic illness after having a baby.

prostaglandin – natural hormones that are involved in many body processes, including pain, tissue injury and inflammation.

psychiatrist – a medically qualified doctor who specialises in mental disorders.

psychiatry – the medical speciality that deals with the management and treatment of mental disorders.

psychoanalysis – a talking therapy based on the teachings of Sigmund Freud.

psychodynamic psychotherapy – one of the talking therapies.

psychologist (clinical) – a non-medically qualified specialist in mental science.

psychology – the study of the way that the mind works.

psychosis – a serious mental disorder in which there may be detachment from reality.

psychotherapist – a practitioner of one of the talking therapies who may or may not be medically qualified.

reflexology – complementary therapy that involves a specific type of massage and manipulation of various reflex areas on the hands and feet.

SAD or Seasonal Affective Disorder – a form of depression that occurs in winter and which responds to light exposure.

self-harm – the deliberate harming of oneself, ranging from minor scratching to cutting and real intent to injure or kill oneself.

suicide – the act of ending one's own life.

suicidal thoughts – thoughts about ending one's life.

Reiki – a complementary therapy alleged to stimulate natural healing.

serotonin – one of the neurotransmitters.

unipolar depression – when there is only depression, without any mania.

Treatment-resistant Depression – sometimes referred to as treatment-refractory depression, it is depression that seems to fail to respond to two courses of antidepressants.

transactional analysis – one of the talking therapies.

voice movement therapy – a therapy that is used to help the individual find their voice to get in touch with their feelings.

yoga – a system of exercises performed to promote control of body and mind.

Directory of useful addresses

Action Postpartum Psychosis Network

The APP Network is a network of women across the UK who have experienced postpartum psychosis, in collaboration with academic experts from Birmingham and Cardiff Universities. Among other things they can offer leaflets and information for women and their families, an online PPtalk forum where women and families can talk with women who have suffered from it, and a peer support network where contacts can be suggested.

Address: FREEPOST RSGT-YJEY-ZRREE Action on Postpartum Psychosis
Room 225 Monmouth House
Department of Psychological Medicine
University Hospital Wales
Heath Park
Cardiff CF14 4XW
Tel: 02920 742 038
Email: app@app-network.org
Website: www.app-network.org/

Alliance of Registered Homeopaths

This is an organisation for professionally qualified homeopaths. A free copy of the ARH Register of qualified homeopaths can be obtained via post, telephone or email.

Address: Millbrook
Millbrook Hill
Nutley
East Sussex TN22 3PJ
Tel/Fax: 01825 714506
Email: info@a-r-h.org

Association for Dance Movement Psychotherapy UK (ADMP UK)

For their directory of therapists see www.admt.org.uk.

Association for Postnatal Illness (APNI)

This association provides a telephone helpline, information and leaflets for sufferers from postnatal illness and a network of volunteers who have suffered from postnatal illness.

Address: 145 Dawes Road
Fulham
London SW6 7EB
Tel: 020 7386 0868
Fax: 020 7386 8885

British Association for Counselling and Psychotherapy (BACP)

The BACP is a membership organisation and a registered charity that sets standards for therapeutic practice and provides information for therapists, clients of therapy, and the general public.

Address: BACP House
15 St John's Business Park
Lutterworth

Leicestershire LE17 4HB
Email: bacp@bacp.co.uk
Website: www.bacp.co.uk

Benefit Enquiry Line

The Benefit Enquiry Line provides advice and information for disabled people and carers on the range of benefits available, including Attendance Allowance, Disability Living Allowance, Carer's Allowance and Carer's Credit.

Address: 2nd Floor
Red Rose House
Lancaster Road
Preston
Lancashire PR1 1HB
Tel: 0800 882 200
Textphone: 0800 243 355 (Monday to Friday, 8 a.m. to 6 p.m.)
Website: www.gov.uk/benefit-enquiry-line

British Association of Art Therapists (BAAT)

For their directory of therapists:

Tel: 020 7686 4216
Website: www.baat.org

British Association of Dramatherapists (BADth)

For their directory of drama therapists:

Tel: 01242 235 515
Website: www.badth.org.uk

British Association for Music Therapy (BAMT)

For information on music therapy in the UK:

Tel: 020 7837 6100

Website: www.bamt.org

British Acupuncture Council

The leading body for the practice of traditional acupuncture in the UK. Their website has a useful 'find a practitioner' function.

Website: www.acupuncture.org.uk

British Medical Acupuncture Society

An association of medical practitioners, nurses, midwives, physiotherapists and dentists, trained in Western Medical Acupuncture. The website has a useful 'find a practitioner' function.

Website: www.medical-acupuncture.co.uk

Childline

This is a national helpline for young people. It can help with all sorts of problems from self-harm to the reporting of sexual abuse.

Tel: 0800 1111

Cry-sis

A helpline offering self-help advice and support to parents with excessively crying and demanding babies.

Tel: 08451 228 669 (9 a.m. to 10 p.m., 7 days a week)

Depression Alliance

While they do not currently run a helpline, you can request an information pack with information about local groups, as well as their letter or email pen-friend scheme, from:

Address: 20 Great Dover Street
London SE1 4LX
Tel: 0845 123 23 20
Email: information@depressionalliance.org

Depression UK

This is a national self-help organisation that helps people cope with depression. It offers friendly, mutual support and advice about self-help. There are pen- and phone-friend services and a D-UK Chat.

Address: c/o Self Help Nottingham
Ormiston House
32–36 Pelham Street
Nottingham NG1 2EG
Email: info@depressionuk.org

Faculty of Homeopathy

The Faculty of Homeopathy promotes the academic and scientific development of homeopathy and ensures the highest standards in the education, training and practice of homeopathy by statutorily registered healthcare professionals. This includes doctors, dentists, nurses, veterinary surgeons, midwives, pharmacists and podiatrists, all of whom have taken further training in homeopathy. There are different grades of membership, from primary certification to specialist accreditation.

Address: Hahnemann House
29 Park Street West
Luton LU1 3BE
Tel: 01582 408680

International Association for Voice Movement Therapy

For their directory of registered practitioners, visit www.iavmt.org.

Mind

Offering help and information about mental health problems.

Address: 15–19 Broadway
Stratford
London E15 4BQ
Tel: 020 8519 2122
Email: contact@mind.org.uk
Helpline/Infoline: 0300 123 3393

For Mind Cymru:

3rd Floor, Quebec House
Castlebridge
5–19 Cowbridge Road East
Cardiff CF11 9AB
Tel: 029 2039 5123
Email: contactwales@mind.org.uk

NHS Direct

This is part of the NHS. You can telephone at any time, 24 hours a day, seven days a week, with a concern and speak to an operator who will take details and will then hand you on to a relevant person who can provide help. You may be advised of another service to contact in their locality. Please note that this service is gradually being replaced by NHS 111 from 2013 onwards.

Tel: 0845 4647 / 111

NICE (National Institute for Health and Care Excellence)

NICE was originally set up in 1999 to reduce variation in availability and quality of NHS treatment and care. NICE issues evidence-based guidance on the management of various conditions and public health guidance recommending best ways to encourage healthy living, promote wellbeing and prevent disease.

Website: www.nice.org.uk

PANDAS

An online community supporting people with antenatal and postnatal depression. They can provide support via a call line, email, or a letter service for those who prefer to express themselves in writing, and can put you in touch with a support group.

Tel: 0843 2898 401
Website: www.pandasfoundation.org.uk

The Reflexology Forum

The Reflexology Forum is the developing regulatory body in the UK for reflexology. There are several organisations which are affiliated with it, including the Association of Reflexologists, British Reflexology Association, the Clinical Association of Reflexologists and the International Federation of Reflexologists.

Address: Dalton House
60 Windsor Avenue
London SW19 2RR
Tel: 0800 037 0130
Email: pr@reflexologyforum.org

The Reiki Association

This is a community of people interested in Reiki. The website gives information about the method.

Website: www.reikiassociation.org.uk

Relate

Relate offers advice, relationship counselling, sex therapy, workshops, mediation, consultations and support face-to-face, by phone and through their website.

Tel: 0300 100 1234
Website: www.relate.org.uk

Rethink Mental Illness

This is a campaigning charity that works with people who have a mental illness, their relatives and friends. It runs mental health services, support groups and an advice and information service.

Tel: 0300 5000 927
Website: www.rethink.org

Royal College of Psychiatrists

The professional body for UK psychiatrists. Their website provides many useful leaflets.

Website: www.rcpsych.ac.uk

Samaritans

This is a registered charity, which offers support to anyone in emotional distress. It is non-religious and apolitical. The service offered is predominantly through telephone calls, but a confidential email service is also provided. You can call 24/7 and you do not have to be suicidal to call.

Address: Freepost RSRB-KKBY-CYJK
Chris, PO Box 90 90
Stirling FK8 2SA
Tel: 08457 90 90 90
Email: jo@samaritans.org

The Society of Homeopaths

The Society of Homeopaths is the largest organisation registering professional homeopaths in Europe.

Address: 11 Brookfield
Duncan Close
Moulton Park
Northampton NN3 6WL
Tel: 0845 450 6611
Email: info@homeo-soh.org

The Silent Cry

This is a charity that was set up in 2008 to help people deal with self-harm and depression. The website has videos and downloadable information.

Address: 1 Milton Hall Road
Gravesend
Kent DA12 1QN
Website: www.thesilentcry.co.uk

UK Council for Psychotherapy (UKCP)

The UKCP holds the national register of psychotherapists, psychotherapists qualified to work with children and young people and psychotherapeutic counsellors, listing those practitioner members who meet exacting standards and training requirements.

Address: 2nd Floor, Edward House
2 Wakley Street
London EC1V 7LT
Tel: 020 7014 9955
Email: info@ukcp.org.uk

YoungMinds

This is a charity committed to improving emotional wellbeing and mental health of children and young people. It runs a Parents' Helpline and online resources that may be very useful.

Parent helpline: 0808 802 5544
Website: www.youngminds.org.uk

References

1 Simon C, Everitt H, Birtwistle J, Stevenson B. *Oxford Handbook of General Practice*, OUP, 2003.

2 Bostwick JM, Pankratz VS. Affective disorders and suicide risk: a reexamination. *Am J Psychiatry* 2000; 157(12):1925–1932.

3 Kulkarni J. Depression as a side effect of the contraceptive pill. *Expert Opin Drug Saf*. 2007; 6(4): 371–374.

4 Schildkraut J. The catecholamine hypothesis of affective disorders: a review of supporting evidence. *Am J Psychiatry* 1965; 122:509–522.

5 Pasco JA, et al. Clinical implications of the cytokine hypothesis of depression; the association between use of statins and aspirin and the risk of major depression. *Psychother and Psychosom* 2010; 79: 323–325.

6 Haeffel GJ, Getchell M, Koposov RA, Yrigollen CM, Deyoung CG, Klinteberg BA et al. Association between polymorphisms in the dopamine transporter gene and depression: evidence for a gene-environment interaction in a sample of juvenile detainees. *Psychol Sci* 2008; 19: 62–69.

7 Kroenke K, Spitzer RL, Williams JB. The PHQ-9: validity of a brief depression severity measure. *J Gen Intern Med* 2001; 16(9): 606–613.

8 Kroenke K, Spitzer RL. The PHQ-9: a new depression and diagnostic severity measure. *Psychiatric Annals* 2002; 32: 509–521.

9 Lancaster CA, Gold KA, Flynn HA, Yoo H, Marcus SM, Davis MM. Risk factors for depressive symptoms during pregnancy: a systematic review. *Am J Obstet Gynecol* 2010; 202(1): 5–14.

10 Wiles N et al. Cognitive behavioural therapy as an adjunct to pharmacotherapy for primary care based patients with treatment resistant depression: results of the CoBalT randomised controlled trial. *Lancet* 2013; 381; 9864: 375–384.

11 Mendlewicz J, Kriwin P, Oswald P, Souery D, Alboni S, Brunello N. Shortened onset of action of antidepressants in major depression using acetylsalicylic acid augmentation: a pilot open-label study. *Int Clin Psychopharmacol* 2006; 21(4): 227–231.

12 Lopez AD, Mathers CD, Ezzati M, Jamison DT, Murray CJ. Global and regional burden of disease and risk factors, 2001: systematic analysis of population health data. *Lancet* 2006; 367(9524): 1747–1757.

13 Almudena Sánchez-Villegas ET, Jokin de Irala MR-C, Pla-Vidal J, Martínez-González MA. Fast-food and commercial baked goods consumption and the risk of depression. *Public Health Nutr* 2012; 15: 424–432. DOI: 10.1017/S1368980011001856.

14 *Public Library of Science*. Eating poorly can make you blue: trans-fats increase risk of depression, while olive oil helps avoid risk. ScienceDaily, 26 Jan. 2011. Web. 13 Feb. 2013.

15 Tolmunen T, Hintikka J, Ruusunen A, Voutilainen S, Tanskanen A, Valkonen VP, et al. Dietary folate and the risk of depression in Finnish middle-aged men. A prospective follow-up study. *Psychother Psychosom* 2004; 73: 334–339.

16 Chishti P, Stone DH, Corcoran P, Williamson E, Petridou E; EUROSAVE Working Group. Suicide mortality in the European Union. *Eur J Public Health* 2003; 13(2): 108–114.

17 Sánchez-Villegas A, Delgado-Rodríguez M, Alonso A, Schlatter J, Lahortiga F, Serra Majem L, Martínez-González MA. Association of the Mediterranean dietary pattern with the incidence of depression: the Seguimiento Universidad de Navarra/University of Navarra follow-up (SUN) cohort. *Arch Gen Psychiatry* 2009; 66(10): 1090–1098.

18 Brunner E, Stallone D, Juneja M, Bingham S, Marmot M. Dietary assessment in Whitehall II: comparison of 7 day diet diary and food-frequency questionnaire and validity against biomarkers. *Br J Nutr* 2001; 86: 405–414.

19 Dowrick C, Ayuso-Mateos JL, Vazquez-Barquero JL, Dunn G, Dalgard OS, Lehtinen V, Casey P, Wilkinson C, Page H, Lasa L, Michalak EE, Wilkinson G; the ODIN Group. From epidemiology to intervention for depressive disorders in the general population: the ODIN study. *World Psychiatry* 2002; 1(3): 169–174.

20 Byrd-Bredbenner C, Lagiou P, Trichopoulou A. A comparison of household food availability in 11 countries. *J Hum Nutr Diet* 2000; 13(3): 197–204.

21 Folkins CH. Effects of physical training on mood. *J Clin Psychol* 1976; 32(2): 385–388.

22 Dimeo F, Bauer M, Varahram I, Proest G, Halter U. Benefits from aerobic exercise in patients with major depression: a pilot study. *Br J Sports Med* 2001; 35(2): 114–117.

23 Blumenthal JA, Babyak MA, Moore KA, Craighead WE, Herman S, Khatri P, Waugh R, Napolitano MA, Forman LM, Appelbaum M, Doraiswamy PM, Krishnan KR. Effects of exercise training on older patients with major depression. *Arch Intern Med* 1999; 159(19): 2349–2356.

24 Dunn AL, Trivedi MH, Kampert JB, Clark CG, Chambliss HO. Exercise treatment for depression: efficacy and dose response. *Am J Prev Med* 2005; 28(1):1–8.

25 Dwivedi Y. Brain-derived neurotrophic factor: role in depression and suicide. *Neuropsychiatr Dis Treat* 2009; 5: 433–449.

26 Hansen CJ, Stevens LC, Coast JR. Exercise duration and mood state: how much is enough to feel better? *Health Psy* 2001; 20(4): 267–275.

27 Lee RE, Goldberg JH, Sallis JF, Hickmann SA, Castro CM, Chen AH. A prospective analysis of the relationship between walking and mood in sedentary ethnic minority women. *Women Health* 2001; 32(4): 1–15.

28 Erkkilä J, Punkanen M, Fachner J, et al. Individual music therapy for depression: randomised controlled trial. *Brit J Psychiat* 2011; 199: 132–139.

29 Streeter CC, Jensen JE, Perlmutter RM, Cabral HJ, Tian H, Terhune DB, Ciraulo DA, Renshaw PF. Yoga Asana sessions increase brain GABA levels: a pilot study. *J Alt Comp Med* 2007; 13(4): 419–426.

30 Streeter CC, Whitfield TH, Owen L, Rein T, Karri SK, Yakhkind A, Perlmutter R, Prescot A, Renshaw PF, Ciraulo DA, Jensen JE. Effects of yoga versus walking on mood, anxiety, and brain GABA levels: a randomized controlled MRS study. *J Alter Comp Med* 2010; 16(11): 1145–1152.

Have you enjoyed this book?
If so, why not write a review on your favourite website?

If you're interested in finding out more about our books,
find us on Facebook at **Summersdale Publishers** and
follow us on Twitter at **@Summersdale.**

Thanks very much for buying this Summersdale book.

www.summersdale.com